YOGA

FOR YOU

YOGA
FOR YOU

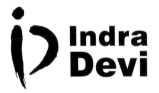

Indra Devi

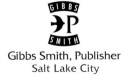

Gibbs Smith, Publisher
Salt Lake City

06 05 04 03 02   5 4 3 2 1

Originally published by Prentice Hall Inc. in 1959 as *Yoga for Americans*
© 1959 Prentice Hall Inc.
© 1959 Editorial Diana S.A.
© 1988 Coedicion de Editorial Diana S.A., y Javier Vergara Editor S.A.
© 1999 Ediciones B Argentina S.A.

Published by
Gibbs Smith, Publisher
P.O. Box 667
Layton, Utah 84041

Orders: (1-800) 748-5439
www.gibbs-smith.com

Printed and bound in Hong Kong

The exercises in this book are gentle and safe provided the instructions are followed
carefully. However, the publisher and authors disclaim all liability in connection with use
of the information in individual cases. If you have any doubts as to the suitability of the
exercises, consult a doctor.

Library of Congress Cataloging-in-Publication Data

Devi, Indra, b. 1899.
  Yoga for you / Fundacion Indra Devi and David Lifszyc.— 1st ed.
    p. cm.
  ISBN 1-58685-141-1
  1. Yoga—Health aspects. I. Lifszyc, David. II. Fundacion Indra Devi.
III. Title.
  RA781.7 .D484 2002
  613.7'046—dc21
                        2001007447

To my friend and pupil
GLORIA SWANSON

For her ever-searching, burning,
crusading spirit, admirable courage,
keen sense of humor and luminous laughter.

CONTENTS

Introduction to the Present Edition x

Concise Biography of Indra Devi xii

The Indra Devi Foundation xxii

Foreword by Yehudi Menuhin xxiii

Author's Preface: How Yoga Can Be of Help to You xxiv

Words of Acknowledgment .xxx

What You Should Know About Yoga xxxi

Lesson One: First Week 41

What the Course Is and How to Use It 41

The Waking-up Routine 42

Deep Breathing 44

Exercises for the Neck and Eyes 51

Yoga Postures 59

    Rocking 60

    Raised Legs Posture (Uddhita Padasana) 62

    Head-to-Knee Posture (Janushirshasana) 64

    Lotus Pose (Padmasana) 66

    Cobra Pose (Bhujanghasana) .69

    Squatting Pose (Utkasana) 70

Breathing Exercises 73

Relaxation 74

General Rules and Recommendations 77

Discussion: On the Effects of Breathing 80

Lesson Two: Second Week 89

The Half-Headstand (Ardha Shirshasana) 92

The Symbol of Yoga (Yoga Mudra) 94

Body-Raising Pose (Ardha Navasana) 96

Bending-Forward Posture (Hastapadasana) 97

Footlift Pose (Ardha Baddha Pada Uttanasana):

First Movement 98

Reverse Posture (Viparita Karani Mudra) 99

Breathing Exercises 102

Rhythmic Breathing 103

Posture for Meditation 105

The Diet 107

Lesson Three: Third Week 127

Headstand (Shirshasana): First Stage 127

Stretching Posture (Paschimotanasana) 131

Plough Posture (Halasana) 134

Camel Posture (Ustrasana) 136

Lion Posture (Simhasana) 137

Footlift Pose (Ardha Baddha Pada Uttanasana):

Second Movement 139

Breathing Exercises 140

Relaxation 142

The Endocrine Glands 146

Lesson Four: Fourth Week .151

Headstand (Shirshasana): Second Stage 152

Swan Posture (Swanasana) 154

Twist Posture (Matsyendrasana): First Movement 156

Abdominal Lift (Uddhiyana Bandha) 158

Churning Pose (Nauli) 160

Footlift Pose (Ardha Baddha Pada Uttanasana):
Third Movement 161
Breathing Exercises 162
Discussion: On the Power of Kundalini 164
The Location of the Chakras 167

Lesson Five: Fifth Week 173
Headstand (Shirshasana): Third Stage 173
Triangle Pose (Upavishta Konasana) 176
Twist Posture (Matsyendrasana): Second Movement 177
Shoulder Stand (Sarvangasana) 178
Supine Pelvic Pose (Supta Vajrasana) 180
Breathing Exercises 181
Discussion: On the Yama-Niyama and Contemplation 184

Lesson Six: Sixth Week 195
Practice Schedule 196
Angular Rest Pose (Supta Konasana) 198
Angular Balance Pose (Urdhva Konasana) 199
Twist Posture (Matsyendrasana): Third Movement 200
Breathing Exercises 201
Discussion: On Concentration and Meditation 204

Appendix I: A Guide to Diet and Recipes 217
The Hay Diet Food Classification .219
Cleansing Diet 222
Health Diet 223
Reducing Diet 224
Diet for People over Thirty-five 224
Recipes 226

**Appendix II: Letters and E-mails to the Author
and to the Indra Devi Foundation** 237

Introduction to the Present Edition

Indra Devi always says that Yoga helps us develop our physical, mental and spiritual well-being in a well-balanced way. Like society, individuals go through permanent change and Yoga is there to help you adapt to these changes. As a science and practical way of life it also evolves and accompanies us during our path through time.

Indra Devi first became a Yoga teacher in the Sri Krishnamacharya tradition in 1939, and until her death at age 102, she still passed on her wisdom and love to thousands. Through the foundation that bears her name, Mataji Indra Devi's teachings are available to all those who wish to practice this way of life.

Our aim is to show you in this new edition of *Yoga for You* the work we are undergoing today at the Indra Devi Foundation. We have reached this point after thoroughly probing and analyzing the experience we have gathered in the last fifteen years and the benefits our students have experienced from our work. However, the core of this book entirely reflects the original one written many years ago by our teacher. Many of the references and books mentioned in this work are out of print, although the reader may come across some of them in secondhand bookstores.

May the Light, the Peace and the Love
Be always present in our path.

Iana and David Lifar
Directors of the Indra Devi Foundation

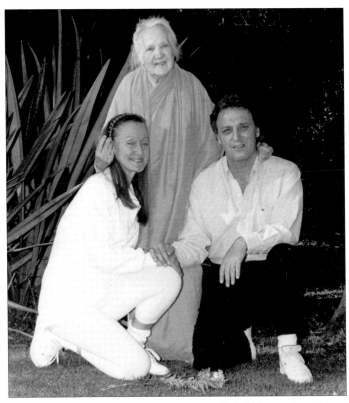

Devi with Iana and David, 1999.

Concise Biography

Mataji Indra Devi, known in the Americas as the "Grande Dame of Yoga," was born Eugenie Peterson in Russia on May 12, 1899. Her mother belonged to the Russian nobility and her father was of Swedish origin. From her youth, Eugenie felt attracted to India, its culture and its spirituality. In 1920, during the civil war, she left Russia with her mother and lived in Germany, where Eugenie joined a famous Russian theater. As a star of this company, she visited most of the European capitals.

Her great dream of going to India was achieved in 1927. She stayed there for twelve years—first as a visitor, then as the wife of a foreign diplomat, and lastly as a Yoga student. Indra Devi, as she was later called, began her Yoga training after being healed by Yogic means of a heart condition that had afflicted her for four years.

While in India, as Mrs. Strakaty, she accomplished many unconventional things, such as playing the first role in an Indian movie and maintaining deep friendships with Pandit Nehru and other fighters for India's freedom. She also met Mahatma Gandhi and the great poet Rabindranath Tagore, among others. She felt happy and equally at ease in a Maharaja's palace as in a humble abode.

Her husband was transferred to China, and, on the advice of her teacher, Shri Krishnamacharya, she opened a Yoga studio in Shanghai in February 1939. Because of her presentations on the stage, Indra Devi also became known as a performer of the Hindu temples' dances, which she had learned in Bombay.

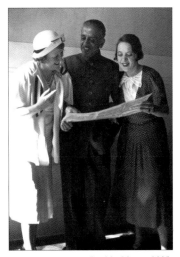

Devi in Mysore, 1935.

After World War I ended, Indra Devi went back to India to continue her advanced Yoga studies in the Himalayas. There, in the heights of the Maharaja of Theri's mountain palace, she wrote her first book, *Yoga,* published in 1948.

Indra Devi began to teach and lecture on this subject, becoming known as the first Westerner to teach Yoga in India. A year later, at the end of 1946, she was called to Shanghai to make use of her belongings. By then, her husband had returned to Europe, where he died.

Instead of returning to India, as she had planned, Indra Devi took a ship to California, where she arrived in January 1947. She soon began to lecture on and teach Yoga in Hollywood. Among her students were Ramón Novarro, Jennifer Jones, Greta Garbo, Robert Ryan, and Gloria Swanson, to whom she dedicated her book *Yoga for Americans.*

Two more books, *Forever Young, Forever Healthy* and *Improve Your Life by Practicing Yoga,* were also published by Prentice Hall in New York. They all soon became best sellers, were translated into ten different languages, and were sold in twenty-nine countries.

In 1953 she married Dr. Sigfrid Knauer, an outstanding physician and a rare humanist. He was a great support to his wife in her job while she was busy teaching, lecturing, issuing TV and radio broadcasts, and conducting press conferences in the United States and in Mexico.

After obtaining American citizenship, which legalized her name as "Indra Devi," she traveled to India, where her book translated into Hindi became known all over the country and even won a government prize as the best nonfiction book.

In 1960, Mataji appeared in international headlines as she presented Yoga to Kremlin officials during a conference organized by the Indian ambassador, K. P. S. Menon. By her explanations to Kosigin, Gromyko, Mikoyan and others about the real meaning of Yoga and its benefits, Mataji caused the prohibition of Yoga to be raised. She was touted by the international press as "the woman who introduced Yoga in the Kremlin."

The following year, her husband bought a beautiful residence in Tecate, Mexico, near the border of California. She established there an international training center for Yoga teachers.

In 1966, she went again to India and also Vietnam in order to lead meditations on the light. During this sojourn at her spiritual home, she met Sathya Sai Baba, worshipped by millions of people all over the world as the avatar of this era.

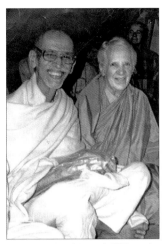

Devi with Swami Chidananda.

From Tecate she traveled twenty-four times to India, moving there
again in 1977, from where she traveled to lecture in the three
Americas. The government of San Salvador invited her to introduce
Yoga in the local schools. It was the first time that a government
understood the huge benefits of Yoga for a complete, total, and integral youth formation.

Mataji Indra Devi went for the first time to Argentina in 1982. In
1985 she decided to stay there, beginning a great work of diffusing
Classic Yoga. She conducted lectures at seminaries in several cities of
Argentina, Brazil, Uruguay, Paraguay, Chile, and Mexico, as well as in
Spain and Germany.

In June 1988, she created *the Indra Devi Foundation, Art and Science
of Living,* which organized the I, II and III Meeting of Yoga
Instructors (April 1988, 1989, 1990), with the presence of Argentine,
American, and European teachers.

In October 1988, she participated in the World Congress that took
place in Uruguay, organized by the Latin American Confederation and
Union of National Yoga Federations (CULFNY). In July 1989, she
was appointed Honorary President of the World Congress in São Paulo,

Brazil, organized by CULFNY, and was specially invited to take part in the Fifth International Conference in February 1990, organized by Unity in Yoga.

In January 1989, she visited her teacher Shri Krishnamacharya, who had reached 100 years of age. In February she visited Mexico, lecturing and conducting spiritual retreats in Cuernavaca.

Between 1990 and 1994, Mataji lectured and taught throughout Germany, Spain, France, England, Russia, India, Mexico, Argentina, and Costa Rica. In the United States, she spread her work through seminars and lectures in Los Angeles, Santa Monica, Portland, Seattle, San Francisco, and Palo Alto.

All through the years, crowds of people and students have approached her to be enlightened by her personal life experiences living intensely and being close to many spiritual leaders. Indra Devi has been one of the most famous teachers who introduced Yoga knowledge and spiritual power in almost all countries of the Americas and continued its spread.

Mataji Indra Devi died April 26, 2002, in Buenos Aires, Argentina, where she had been living. Classic Yoga, as a kind of art and science of life spiritually based on Patanjali's Yoga, was expounded through her teachings. Hers was a unique method for a harmonic and integral development of the human being in his/her physical, mental, and spiritual sides, in order to enjoy a healthy and happy life, with no illness, no tensions, no stress, and above all, with no fear of either life or death.

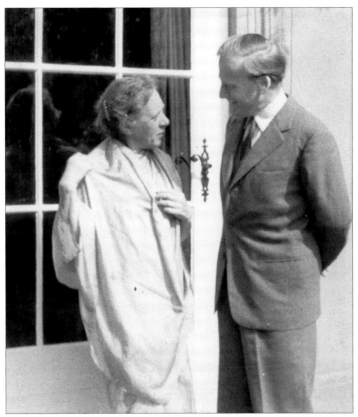

Devi with the famous violinist Yehudi Menuhin in Londres.

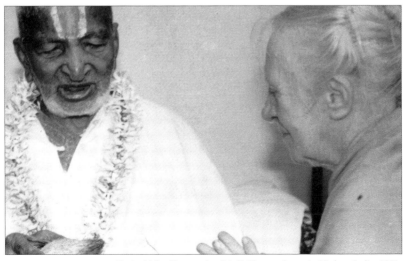

Devi with her Yoga teacher Sri. Krishnamacharya in Madras, India, 1988.

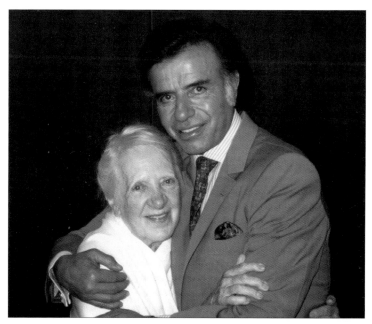

Devi with President Menen in Buenos Aires, 1998.

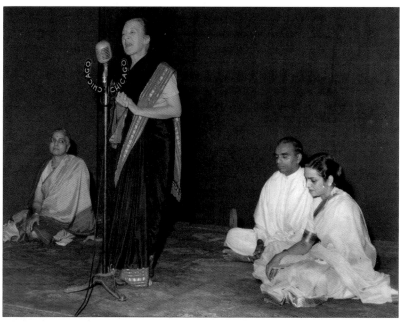

Devi with B.K.S. Iyengar on Radio Chicago in Bombay, 1946.

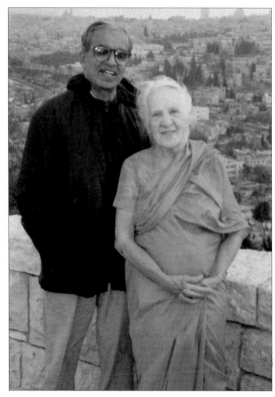

Devi with T.K.V. Desikachar in Jerusalem.

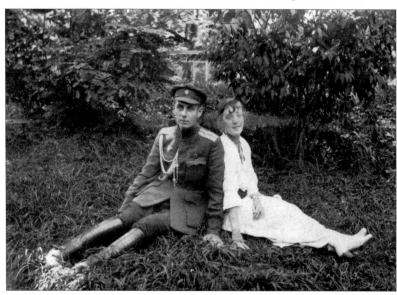

Devi with her boyfriend in Russia, 1917.

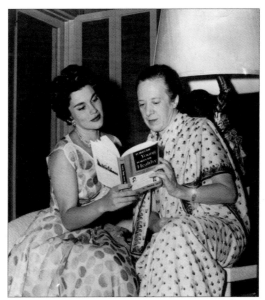

Devi with long-time student Linda Christian (Mrs. Tyrone Power).

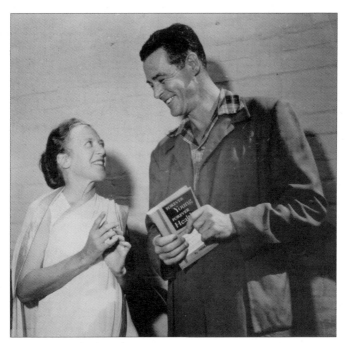

Devi with Robert Ryan.

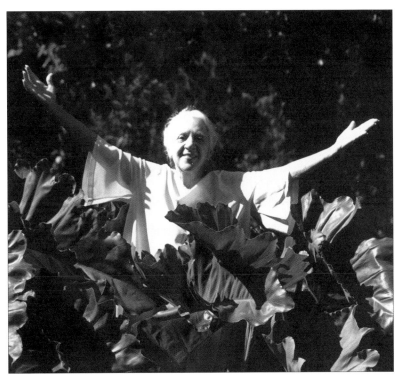

Devi in the garden of her ranch outside of Buenos Aires, Argentina, 1994.

The Indra Devi Foundation

The Indra Devi Foundation was created in March 1988, and today, after ten years of teaching and promoting Yoga, is part of the City of Buenos Aires' Association of Private Organizations. A nonprofit organization, the Foundation's goals are to promote, divulge, motivate, help, participate in and support any kind of program, plan or enterprise that approaches Classic Yoga in an intellectual or educational way, in order to improve the physical, mental and spiritual development of human beings and all their abilities.

Lessons such as Better Breathing for Better Living, Stress Management, Ayurveda, and Total Yoga, added to the classic course options, are the result of the study, experience and evolution that takes place naturally within the Foundation. Today Yoga is available as an instrument to the society as a whole, and it is our wish that you know about us and get involved in this practice, as it will allow you to live a healthier, fuller and more balanced life.

Please visit us at www.fundacion-indra-devi.org.

Foreword

This welcome book by Indra Devi is further evidence of the interest that has been awakened in the United States and other countries of the Western world for the practical aspects of the ancient science of Yoga, and for their application to our own way of living.

Yoga is one of the greatest disciplines in the world and can be practiced at each stage with positive results. It aims at controlling one's spiritual and mental climate. The circulation of the blood, the degree of tension in the muscles and in the nerves, the very thoughts that enter the mind—all of these are subject to progressive control.

The achievement of the final stage of bliss is beyond the conception of most mortals, even yogis themselves, and is reached only by a few who have passed through all the stages and have proven themselves worthy by their own merits.

I can recommend Yoga wholeheartedly from my own experience. It is an unfailing source of vitality and good humor.

Let us learn a little of its philosophy and its application, just as India and all the Eastern world today are busy learning what we know and what we can teach.

Yehudi Menuhin

Author's Preface
How Yoga Can Be of Help to You

To be honest, I did not intend to write again on Yoga postures, since my previous book, *Forever Young, Forever Healthy,* had already described them and spoken at length on relaxation, breathing, diet, weight control and such common complaints as tension, nervousness, insomnia, colds, headaches, constipation, asthma, arthritis, etc. In fact, I did not think that another book on this subject would be necessary. However, since moving to Argentina, I have worked intensely on everything that relates to this art and science of life, to which I have dedicated most of my existence.

During this new period that began in February 1985, I started to realize how important it was to update the books that I had written many years ago. In this my latest edition I have tried to explain step by step, in a more clear and didactic way, with the aid of graphs and pictures, each of the new postures, especially to those who are beginners in Yoga.

There were many people who were hoping for a more detailed program of activities that they could practice every day, both in Argentina and in other countries. They were convinced that once it was available, they would experience, as beginners, more confidence in what they were doing and also feel that they were coached and taught, without being left to their own devices.

Many were also afraid of falling into the hands of charlatans and self-appointed teachers when seeking advice, since there seems to be quite a number of unscrupulous and dishonest individuals who call themselves yogis, but who are really only out to exploit Yoga.

The desire to give a clearer understanding of Yoga and the possibility of studying its health methods at home were what actually spurred me on in writing this book, as well as learning of the shocking state of health in many countries, where physical and mental illness statistics are ever increasing and the number of alcoholics, narcotic addicts, delinquents and criminals is growing at an alarming rate.

It seems to me that, instead of trying to conquer space, it would be better to mobilize the resources countries count on to make sure that the number of able-bodied and mentally sound people does not continue shrinking. Undoubtedly, there must be ways of preventing such a possible disaster if one earnestly decides to do something about it.

I feel very confident that if the study of Yoga were to be added to the curricula of our schools, colleges and physical education programs, it would help considerably in decreasing the menacing incidence of physical and mental disorders. A step toward this goal was taken in San Salvador in January 1986, when I was invited by the government in this Central American country to teach a course for physical education professors, which was also taped so that it could be later utilized as didactic material. Brazil has also made progress in this matter, as I was able to appreciate in the Congress for the International Federation of Yoga Professors and Institutes, in November of 1987, which took place in Montevideo, Uruguay, where they acknowledged the right to teach extracurricular courses for becoming a Yoga instructor at official and religious universities. And in Argentina, the Indra Devi Foundation has been officially authorized to train Yoga instructors, in addition to teaching classes for children, young people, and adults.

The science of Yoga has a separate area devoted to the thorough care of the human body and all of its functions, from breathing to excretion. Its methods are entirely different from other methods of health education, because Yoga aims, first of all, at removing the very causes of illness that are brought about by insufficient oxygenation, poor nutrition, inadequate exercise and poor elimination of the waste products that poison the system. But, also, Yoga can contribute to the increase of mental capacities, as well as sharpen our senses and widen our intellectual horizon through rhythmic breathing and concentration, as well as influencing glandular activity. Finally, through meditation, it enables man to come closer to the realization of his own spiritual nature.

In short, Yoga can help solve the problems of any receptive individual, whether these problems be of physical, mental, or spiritual nature, and, thereby, eventually help solve the problems of a group, society and even a country as well.

Having realized the many advantages of Yoga, the government of India is beginning to encourage the practice of Asanas, or Yoga postures, on a nationwide scale. Thus, for example, toward the late fifties in Delhi, Asanas were being taught to people in all walks of life, regardless of their activity or social class. Early in the morning, open-air instruction was offered in public parks or other public places; and special classes were even conducted for members of Parliament. The Prime Minister in those times was a great Yoga enthusiast and attributed his energy and youthfulness to the daily practice of Asanas, especially of the Headstand. He once made a statement to that effect to newspaper reporters who interviewed him during one of his visits to Japan, which prompted the Japanese publishers of my book, *Forever Young, Forever Healthy*—the first book on Yoga published in Japanese, as I am told— to include his picture and statement on the cover. Unfortunately, the situation in India today is completely different from what it used to be when I first arrived in this country many years ago.

On the other hand, while recovering from his illness, President Eisenhower himself was put on a routine of "deep breathing" exercises for ten minutes a day, according to newspaper reports. But this fact slipped by unnoticed, probably because no formal mention of Yoga was made in connection to it. A real shame, since the publishing of an article on this issue might have started a trend for deep breathing in America— since the public in general likes to imitate the tastes and habits of its leaders and idols. Thus, a great many people seemed to have taken up the study of Yoga simply because it came to be known that it was practiced by such stars as Gloria Swanson, Greta Garbo, Jennifer Jones, Marilyn Monroe, Olivia de Havilland, Mala Powers, Robert Ryan and even the once world-celebrated Elizabeth Arden, a specialist in beauty items. Imagine, then, how people would have been influenced in the United States by the breathing practices of their president!

I have been able to understand how great an influence advocacy by a known personality may have on the public through my own personal experience. Thus, for example, after one of my lectures in which I mentioned Gloria Swanson, I was asked more questions about the actress than about Yoga itself, which did not prevent favorable changes from occurring, since Gloria's enthusiasm for Yoga helped a great deal in making Yoga popular in this country. And when she introduced my book—and me—to the audience attending my opening lecture at the Waldorf Astoria Hotel in New York, she stated unequivocally that Yoga was her health and beauty secret.

The great violinist Yehudi Menuhin considered Yoga—and sleep—to be even more important to his art than violin practice, according to an article in *Life* magazine. His Yoga instructor in India, B. K. S. Iyengar of Poona, wore a wristwatch inscribed, "To my best violin teacher . . . from Yehudi Menuhin."

Yoga is of great value not only to artists engaged in creative work, but to people in business and sports, to public speakers, models and housewives, and also to people employed in offices, factories and stores whether they have to sit at a desk, stand on their feet for long hours at a time, or work under stress and tension.

In his article "Deep Breathing Advised to Alleviate Heart Pain," George W. Crane, M.D., Ph.D., states that the "deep breathing" technique is an excellent aid in every case of sudden heart attack, regardless of its type. "Simply lie flat, relax, breathe deeply, and let God carry on."[1]

Dr. Fedor Stefanovich, who introduced a procedure in Mexico for women to give birth in a natural and painless way, was so enthusiastic about Yoga breathing and its relaxation methods that he decided to include them in his program.

The same course of action was followed by Dr. Rafael Ramos Méndez, a truly remarkable man who directs a school for educating and rehabilitating children who have suffered poliomyelitis' consequences, and to whom he educates, instructs, feeds and gives free medical treatment with orthopedic devices.

While in Mexico, I was also visited by a pilot who assured me that Yoga exercises and deep breathing had helped him so much in his life and activities that he sent a letter to all his fellow pilots, encouraging them to practice Yoga to improve their skills as pilots.

In Argentina, where I have lived since 1982, I have seen many examples of how Yoga helped to change the life of thousands of people. I have been fortunate to accompany these changes, thanks to the teaching we offer at my Foundation centers, where we faithfully convey the essential principles of Yoga, from the most basic act of breathing, to the benefits of the Asanas, the learning of relaxation in the middle of a world that is so stressed, and the initiation in the practice of meditation.

Yoga exercises are, incidentally, an invaluable aid to keeping a trim and youthful figure, and many people will find them effective in helping to solve their physical problems.

The six-week course that is outlined in these pages is organized in such a manner that even someone who has never done any exercises or has never even heard of Yoga will have no difficulty in following it.

Yoga gives forth a message that is full of hope and is practical for our restless, insecure, and spiritually deprived world of today. I truly hope that these lessons will be at least of some small service to those who strive for a better, healthier, and happier life.

Mataji Indra Devi

1. *Glendale News-Press,* December 7, 1955.

Words of Acknowledgment

My grateful thanks to my best friend and guide, Dr. Sigfrid Knauer, for his understanding, cooperation, and advice; and to Dr. Ehrenfried E. Pfeiffer, for the privilege of letting me use material from the manuscript of his work *Balanced Nutrition—Know What You Eat and Why*.

I am also indebted to my friends Erica Moore, for her invaluable help in getting this manuscript into shape; Maurine Dudley Townsend, for putting the finishing touches to it; and Therese Voelker, for her devoted patience in copying it from my hieroglyphic handwriting.

Lastly, my most heartfelt gratitude to Iana and David Lifar, for their unconditional companionship and support since coming to live in Argentina. They have received my legacy with unfailing spirit and have taken charge of the Foundation that carries my name and is committed to passing on the teachings of my mentors, as significant to today's world as they were for me many years ago.

What You Should Know About Yoga

Welcome, friend, to the ever-growing circle of Yoga students in the United States, as well as the world over. I hope that the study and practice of this most ancient, yet still unsurpassed, art and science of living will give you the key to youth, health and long life, and help you find harmony, peace of mind and true happiness. Yoga has been doing so for countless people throughout the centuries, and it is now your turn to try this ancient method and test its effectiveness. For, unless you yourself are benefited by Yoga, no retelling of even the most wonderful results achieved by others will be of the slightest use to you.

Once you start to practice the Yoga lessons, you will experience the benefits in your everyday life. You will begin to enjoy better health, sounder sleep, a keener mind and a more cheerful disposition. Your body will gradually acquire a pleasant lightness and suppleness, your mind will become calmer and your tensions diminish. You will also notice an improvement in your figure, posture, vision, and general appearance, for you will start looking younger and feeling more alive.

The secret of Yoga lies in the fact that it deals with the entire human being, not with just one of his or her aspects. It is concerned with growth—physical, mental, moral and spiritual. It develops forces that are already within you. Beginning with improved health and added physical well-being, it works up slowly through the mental to the spiritual. The transition is so gradual that you may not even be aware of it until you realize that a change in you has already taken place.

The following passage from a work on Yoga will explain how this actually happens:

When a student of Yoga determines and rightly directs his course, a molecular change takes place in his body until, in about six months, this change begins to affect his tastes and habits. It also expands the power of his mind. As the force within him becomes awakened, his state of consciousness also changes—he ceases to be lonely, his fears vanish and his happiness comes within his reach.

The advanced stages of Yoga require many years of special preparation, based on rigorous practices for which the American way of life, its pace and surroundings, are not well suited. Under the existing circumstances, these advanced practices may even prove dangerous and detrimental to the physical and mental well-being and balance of the practitioner. Therefore, I suggest you leave them alone and limit yourself to the practice of the Yoga postures and deep breathing and relaxation exercises, devoting some time to concentration and meditation.

Before we begin the important part of our first lesson, the deep breathing and postures, I would like to give you a general idea of what Yoga is in a question and answer form, so that as a student you may begin to understand it. But first, please do not make the mistake so common in the U.S. of using the words yogi and Yoga interchangeably. Yoga is the science that gives a human being the knowledge of his true Self; a yogi is a man who has mastered this science. The woman is a yógini.

Many people still think that Yoga is a religion. Others believe it to be a kind of magic. Some associate Yoga with the rope trick, with snake charming, fire eating or sitting on nail beds, lying on broken glass, walking on sharp swords, etc. Sometimes it is even linked to fortune telling, spiritualism, hypnotism and other "isms." In reality, Yoga is a method, a system of physical, mental and spiritual development.

Q: What is the meaning of the word "Yoga"?

A: The word Yoga derives from the Sanskrit root "yuj," which means to join, or also union. The purpose of all forms of Yoga is to unite man, the finite, with the Infinite, with Cosmic Consciousness, Truth, God, Light or whatever other name one chooses to call the Ultimate Reality. Yoga, as they say in India, is a marriage of spirit and matter.

Q: Is there only one Yoga?

A: Yoga has several branches or divisions, but the goal, the aim of all of them is the same—the achievement of a union with the Supreme Consciousness. In Karma Yoga, for instance, this is achieved through work and action; in Jnana (or Gnani) Yoga, through knowledge and study; in Bhakti Yoga, through devotion and selfless love; in Mantra Yoga, through repetitions of certain invocations and sounds. Raja Yoga (Royal Yoga) is the Yoga of consciousness, the highest form of Yoga. Its practice usually starts with Hatha Yoga, which gives the body the necessary health and strength to endure the hardships of the more advanced stages of training.

Hatha Yoga is the Yoga of physical well-being. It consists of several steps and is preceded by the Yama-Niyama, the ten rules of the Yoga code of morality. The first stage is called Asana, or posture; the second is Pranayama, or breath control; the third is Pratyahara, or nerve control; the fourth is Dharana, or mind control; the fifth is Dhyana, or meditation; and finally there is Samadhi, the state of ultimate bliss and spiritual enlightenment. Strictly speaking, the last four stages of Hatha Yoga already merge into the realm of Raja Yoga.

Q: What does "Hatha" mean?

A: *Ha* stands for sun and *tha* for moon. The correct translation of Hatha Yoga would be solar and lunar Yoga, since it deals with the solar and lunar qualities of breath and Prana.

Q: What is "Prana"?

A: Prana is a subtle life energy existing in the air in fluid form. Everything living, from men to amoebae, from plants to animals, is charged with Prana. Without Prana there is no life.

Q: What religion does a yogi profess?

A: A yogi can belong to any religion or to none at all. In this case, he usually forms his own relationship with the Ultimate Reality once he has come close to It.

Q: Can a Catholic take up Yoga?

A: Certainly, since Yoga is not a religion. In fact, a Catholic association was formed in Bangalore, India, in order to introduce the Yoga Asanas to the Catholic young men there, and to integrate them into the Catholic way of life.

Q: If the goal of Yoga is a spiritual illumination, why then is so much attention given to the care of the body?

A: The yogis regard the human body as a temple of Light and believe that as such it should be brought to the highest state of perfection. Also, the advanced practices of Yoga require great power of endurance, which may not be achieved without special preparation.

Q: What is the origin of Yoga?

A: Yoga was originated in India several thousand years ago. According to the German professor Max Muller, Yoga is about 6,000 years old, but other sources suggest it is much older.

Q: Who was the first to make Yoga known?

A: This is not known. Patanjali, who lived about 200 B.C., is called the Father of Yoga because he was the first to put into writing what had until then been handed down only verbally from master, or *guru*, to pupil, or *chela*.

Q: Can the average Occidental take up Yoga to improve his physical condition?

A: Yoga postures, breathing and relaxation exercises can be taken up by anyone who wants to improve his or her physical or mental condition. Each individual may move on, according to his or her own needs or wishes, to the more advanced stages of Yoga.

Q: What is the age limit for a Yoga student?

A: Normally, one should not start before the age of six nor after the age of seventy-five, although many people do start later and still obtain good results. One can continue the practice of Yoga postures for the rest of one's life.

Q: Can Yoga cure disease?

A: I don't think the question is well formulated. It is nature that does the healing. Yoga exercises can only help remove impurities and obstructions, so that nature may be given a chance to accomplish her task successfully.

Q: What is the difference between Yoga postures and other gym exercises?

A: Yoga Asanas are an art applied to the anatomy of the living body, whereas gymnastics are a form of engineering applied to the muscles of the body. The aim of Yoga postures is not merely the superficial development of muscles. These postures tend to normalize the functions of the entire organism, regulating the involuntary processes of respiration, circulation, digestion, elimination, metabolism, etc., and to affect the working of all the glands and organs, as well as the nervous system and the mind. This result is achieved by doing deep breathing while the body is placed in various postures. Each of these exercises produces a different overall effect in the functional relationships within the organism.

Hence, Yoga is able to influence man physically, mentally, morally and spiritually. Yoga gives a unique importance to the philosophy of exercise. All the individual capacities are heightened, and man achieves balance and stamina through these exercises, some of which are modeled after the movements of various animals. In Yoga, relaxation is considered an art, breathing a science, and mental control of the body a means of harmonizing the body, mind and spirit.

Infinite energy is at the disposal of man
if he knows how to get it, and
this is a part of the science of Yoga.

—ADAMS BECK, The Story of Philosophy

Lesson One • First Week

*Only a few men die from sudden lack of air,
but multitudes perish because for years they
have not been breathing enough.*

—RASMUS ALSAKER, M.D., Master Key Is Health

What This Course Is and How to Use It

As the title of my book implies, the course of exercises outlined here
for home practice is designed to teach the rudiments of Yoga so that
they can be incorporated into the daily routine of the average man or
woman living in the Western world. I have taken into account not
only the pace of life in this part of the world, but also the unquestion-
able fact that most of my readers have not had the chance to keep
their muscles flexible and their joints supple. At first glance, as you go
through the illustrations and pictures in this book, some of the Yoga
poses may seem impossibly difficult to you—and you may feel you
cannot even attempt them. But please don't feel discouraged. If you
follow instructions, with a little patience and method you will be able
to learn a great deal more than you think possible—and in less time
than you imagine.

The course is divided into six lessons. Each lesson consists of a number of breathing exercises and Yoga postures, probably more than you will normally have time for. You will find yourself liking some better than others, and you will want to let your personal preferences guide you when it comes to choosing those you want to incorporate into your own personal routine. Once you have decided, repeat your chosen routine every day for a week, in order to give yourself a chance to assimilate it before going on to the next week's set of instructions. As you practice the same postures day by day, you will find your muscles stretching, your body growing more responsive and in control, until what seemed unattainable on Monday has become routine on Saturday. Then you will be ready to go on to the next week's lesson.

I also want to make clear that throughout the book I have tried, while outlining each day's schedule, to adjust to the regular waking and sleeping hours of the average person. Those who keep odd bed and meal hours will need to adjust this schedule, making whatever changes are necessary in order to suit their particular time requirements. The best time is, of course, in the morning before breakfast, but it does not matter too much at what time of day the exercises are done, as long as they are done on an empty stomach. Allow three to four hours after a big meal, one and a half to two hours after a light meal, and about half an hour after a glass of juice. Neither is it recommended to do the exercises directly before eating. But the most important thing of all is to do them regularly, without skipping any session. If, by any reason, you do not have time for all of them, do just a few, perhaps even only one when you are in a great hurry—but never omit them entirely. Once you begin to skip any, you are likely to fall back into a sedentary way until you stop exercising altogether.

The Waking-Up Routine

We shall begin our first lesson with the routine you should adopt the moment you open your eyes in the morning and are ready to get up.

First of all, learn to wake up properly. Do some stretching. Extend your arms, yawn several times, stretch your legs, stretch your whole body. While you are still in bed, do the following stretching exercise:

Keeping your feet together, toe to toe, start to stretch the right leg, without raising it off the mattress, as if you wanted to lengthen it. The pull should be felt from the hip down and momentarily, the leg will be lengthened by an inch or more. Hold your leg in this position while you count to sixty; then relax, allowing the right foot to become even again with the left one. Repeat with the left leg.

This exercise stretches the spinal column and tones up the sympathetic nerves. It has a rejuvenating effect on the entire body. Because this is a very potent nerve exercise, you must be careful not to overdo it. Sixty seconds for each leg is the maximum. You may, however, repeat the exercise again in the evening if you wish. If your mattress is too soft, don't do this in bed, but wait until you are ready to do the other exercises on the floor and simply begin with this one.

Incidentally, if you want to avoid those all too frequent backaches, don't ever sleep on a soft mattress. Get a hard one or put a board under the soft mattress. Just try it out for a week or so and you will notice the difference in the way you feel. When traveling or staying in hotels, I often pull the mattress down to the floor, unless it is too heavy. If I find I cannot handle the mattress, I slip the glass top from a dressing table under it.

Another important thing to bear in mind is never to rush out of bed, even if you are in a hurry, as this gives the whole nervous system a shock. Give yourself a little time to return to this world from the threshold of another. Make this transition slowly and gradually and give your body time to "shift gears." Animals offer a good example of natural behavior. Watch, for example, a cat or a dog. Except when in danger or an emergency, they never jump up, but keep yawning and stretching for quite a while until they become fully awake; then they slowly get up on their feet. Imitate them.

When you finally get out of bed, drink a glass of water, but make sure it is at room temperature, not iced. Drink it after brushing your teeth and cleaning your tongue with a special tongue scraper or with a washcloth. As you already probably know, the tongue is a barometer that shows the condition of your intestinal tract. A bright red tongue indicates a clean intestinal tract, whereas a coated tongue indicates the opposite. If the latter is the case, you should plan to go on a cleansing diet or fast for a few days to get rid of the impurities accumulated in your body. We shall discuss this at length later on.

Now let us return to the exercises. As already said, they should be done with an empty stomach, empty bladder and also, if possible, empty bowels. When you are all ready to start, put on a minimum of clothing and make sure that whatever you are wearing is comfortable and not tight. Do not wear a bra, tight belt or other close-fitting garments while exercising. You may wear a pair of socks if your feet feel too cold.

Deep Breathing

Yoga gives great importance to our relationship with the universe, and therefore it teaches a breathing that is different from the usual breathing, a breathing that reflects our inner attitude while we are performing it. This attitude is one of devotion, that is, of communion with the All, and should be maintained all the time one is doing deep breathing.

CONSCIOUS BREATHING

I shall begin with an explanation of Yoga breathing, as it is of utmost importance for you to understand, first of all, how this deep breathing is done and how it differs from ordinary breathing.

Usually we are not conscious of our breathing. Breath passes through our bodies like the waves in a dream. In Yoga, this process is lifted to the level of consciousness. It is you yourself who take over the direction and control of the airflow.

In normal respiration the air is taken in through the nostrils without any special effort, or without any exaggerated or forced movement of the nose or chest. In short, it is done unconsciously. We are not even aware of the air traveling through our nostrils, down the nasal and oral parts of the pharynx, into the larynx, until it reaches the trachea and the lungs. Moreover, not only are we unaware of the breathing process, but most of us do not even know anything about it. You can easily prove this for yourself by asking several friends to answer this simple question: "What happens to the air after it enters your nostrils?" They will probably tell you it goes to the lungs, although everybody realizes in a general way that the nose does not reach that far and that there is quite a distance between it and the lungs.

Taking into consideration the limited knowledge we possess about the function of our organism, I will try to make my anatomical explanations as simple as possible. It is very easy to demonstrate the deep-breathing technique, but not nearly as easy to put it in words. We shall therefore go into it in some detail so that you may be able to grasp the idea correctly.

THE ANATOMY OF BREATHING

Let us begin by analyzing the way the so-called Yoga deep-breathing exercise is usually done, and see in what way it differs from ordinary deep breathing.

Take a deep breath. Just put down the book for a moment and do it the way you have always been doing it. Most people vigorously sniff air in through the nostrils, simultaneously raising the chest and popping out the eyes. Well, Yoga deep breathing is not done this way at all. Let us examine what happens when you take the usual kind of deep breath. First of all, you interrupt your normal—or unconscious—breathing and make a conscious and deliberate effort to inhale. In doing this, you use considerable force. You also produce a loud sniffing sound by automatically contracting the nostrils. In Yoga, the process of deep breathing is so entirely different that it is better to completely forget the way you have been doing it up to now.

To begin with, you do not consciously use the nostrils at all; they must remain completely inactive during inhalation and exhalation. Instead, you draw in the air by using the area situated at the back wall of your mouth, called the pharyngeal area. This connects the mouth with the nose, and is the continuation of the nasal openings, which end behind the soft palate leading from the mouth into the throat.

You will understand this even better if you take a hand mirror and look into it to see the back of your mouth. I suggest that since you have already interrupted your reading, you pick up a mirror right now, otherwise you will probably forget about it. What you see, especially as you press down the tongue, is a cave in the form of a dome. The air passage takes place directly beneath this dome. This is the pharyngeal area. And it is this area, and not the nostrils, that you must learn to use in Yoga deep breathing. This, then, is the main technical difference between ordinary deep breathing and Yoga deep breathing. Had you ever been aware before of the possibility of drawing in air through an area other than the nostrils? Probably not. However, people suffering from a post-nasal drip learn perfectly well of this other area.

If you sniff in water, especially salt water, through the nostrils and eject it through the mouth, you will immediately become aware of the pharyngeal area, which connects the mouth with the nose. It is this connection that makes it possible to draw the air in through the pharyngeal area, while keeping the nostrils completely inactive during deep breathing. The action is felt only at the back of the throat during the exhalation and the impression is that of a hydraulic suction pump or press operating in the back of the mouth. In fact, the entire action is similar, since during inhalation one feels as if the air were being drawn in, and during exhalation as if it were being pressed down the throat, though in reality, of course, it is being expelled.

It really should not be too difficult for you to do the deep-breathing routine since you have already been doing it for a long time, and without any instructions. Without your being aware of it, this is exactly what takes place while you are sleeping, for in sleep the sense organism is not functioning and cannot therefore interfere with the rhythm of breathing. When asleep, we automatically, or shall I say instinctively, resort to deep breathing at certain intervals. This probably is an indication that deep breathing is of an elemental nature and we can, by means of it, consciously establish a contact between our inner selves and the deep forces of Nature.

LEARNING TO BREATHE CORRECTLY

Since you know how to do deep breathing while asleep, a simple method of learning to do it during wakefulness should be to simulate sleep. Lie down, close your eyes, relax the whole body, drop the chin and imagine that you are asleep, thus letting your breathing become deeper and deeper. But first, a word of warning: When exaggerated and overstrained, deep breathing leads to snoring, so you'd better learn to relax and breathe softly and gently. Also, the next time you happen to be in a room with someone who is fast asleep, listen for a while to his or her respiration; you will quickly notice the difference, both in sound and rhythm, between the "waking" and the "sleeping" breath.

In Yoga, deep breathing starts by filling the lower part of the lungs first, then the middle and finally the upper part. When exhaling, you first empty the upper part of the lungs, then the middle, and last of all the lower part.

This process, however, should not be thought of as three separate actions. Inhalation is done in one smooth continuous flow just as one might pour water to fill a glass. First the bottom is filled, then the middle, and finally the upper portion. But not because of this sequence is the process of filling the entire glass interrupted. Just so is the air taken in, in one uninterrupted inhalation, while the lungs fill with air; and also the air expelled until the lungs are empty. But you must do it slowly and perfectly relaxed. No effort or strain should ever be exerted. This is very important. Keep mouth closed, as breathing is always done through the nose.

You then become aware of the function of your own diaphragm. When you inhale, it expands your chest, and, when you exhale, it contracts it. The lower part of the rib cage naturally expands first when you breathe in, and is compressed last, when you exhale. This, too, we insist should be done gently, without any force or strain. The chest must remain motionless and passive during the entire process of respiration. Only the ribs expand during inhalation and contract during exhalation, like an accordion. It is a serious mistake to use force during inhalation. It should be done with ease, without any tension or strain whatsoever. In deep breathing, exhalation is as important as inhalation, because it eliminates toxic substances. It is very seldom that the lower part of our lungs are sufficiently emptied, and consequently they tend to accumulate air saturated with waste products, for with ordinary breathing we never expel enough of the carbon dioxide our system throws off, even if we do inhale enough oxygen. Also, when the lower parts of our lungs are properly expanded and contracted, the circulation in the liver and spleen greatly benefits, as they are thus "massaged" by the diaphragm.

Another important thing to remember is that while doing deep breathing the spine should be kept straight, so as not to impair the free flow of the life-force, or Prana. This also helps to develop correct posture. Yogis attach such great importance to correct posture that they have devised several different positions for their various advanced breathing practices as well as for meditation and concentration.

Their favorite posture is the Lotus Pose, or Padmasana, a word derived from Padma, which means lotus in Sanskrit, and Asana, which means posture. (The accent in Padmasana falls on the first syllable of the second word, Asana, not on the second as would be natural in English.) The other three postures are Siddhasana, Swastikasana, and Samasana. You will learn them one by one later on.

In all of these postures, the spine has to be erect, in one straight line with the head, neck and trunk. The need for keeping the spine straight is emphasized in all Yoga practices where it is an important requisite. Only man, the crowning of creation, has acquired a vertical spine, through the awakening of his consciousness; the spine is considered a symbolical connecting link between earth and heaven.

When you sit down on the floor with your legs crossed, visualize a stream running through you in a straight line, starting at the top of your head and continuing into the ground. Imagine, too, that this stream is the axis around which your body has been shaped. This will help you learn to sit up straight without being stiff and tense. You should, in fact, feel comfortable and relaxed as you sit this way.

YOUR FIRST DEEP BREATH

Now, sit down on your exercise mat or rug intended for your practice and get ready to start your first real lesson in deep breathing. If for some reason you are unable to sit on the floor, you may sit on a chair or else stand up. Deep breathing can also be done lying down, provided the spine is kept straight. But normally we should do it while sitting cross-legged. If you cannot assume the Lotus Posture as yet, cross your legs in any way that is easiest for you. (The complete technique for assuming the Lotus Pose is given later in this lesson.)

Again, first check your posture. The spine should be straight, the head erect, hands on knees, mouth closed. Now, concentrate on the pharyngeal space at the back wall of your mouth and, slightly contracting its muscles, begin to draw in the air through that space as if you were using a suction pump. Do it slowly, steadily, letting the pumping sound be clearly heard. Don't use the nostrils; remember that they remain inactive during the entire respiration process. When inhaling, let your ribs expand sideways like an accordion—beginning with the lower ones, of course. Remember the chest and shoulders should remain motionless. The entire inhalation should be done gently and effortlessly. When it has been completed, pause for a second or two, holding your breath. Then slowly begin breathing out. The exhalation is usually not as passive as the inhalation. You use a slight, very slight, pressure to push the air out, although it feels as though you pressed it against the throat like a hydraulic press. The upper ribs are now contracted first, the nostrils remain inactive and the chest and shoulders motionless. At the end of the exhalation, pull in the stomach a little so as to push out all the air.

You have just taken your first deep breath.

The beginner should not try to take too full a breath at once. Start by breathing to the count of four. Then hold the breath, counting to two, and start slowly exhaling, again to the count of four. Breathing in and out to an equal number of beats is called rhythmic breathing, although there are other types of rhythmic breathing where inhaling and exhaling are carried out to different beats.

You should fill your lungs while counting to four, hold your breath while counting to two, and exhale again to the count of four. The respiration should be timed in such a way that at the end of the four beats you have completed the exhalation. Don't just stop at the end of the count when there is still air to be expelled. You should adjust your breathing to the timing. Repeat, but do not take more than 5 or 6 deep breaths at one time during the first week.

This is enough for today. You shouldn't do more even if you are enjoying it. Be careful not to overdo the breathing, especially inhalation, as this may lead to unpleasant results, such as dizziness, nausea, headaches, and even fainting spells, due to hyperventilation caused by a sudden, excessive intake of oxygen. You should not invite unnecessary trouble, but get full benefit from these lessons. As your teacher, it is my duty to warn you against possible ill effects caused by over-breathing. Please be patient; it is for your own good that I am offering this advice.

Deep breathing is often quite a revelation to people who do it for the first time. "I just discovered my lungs," a man once said to me. He happened to be a photographer who came with a reporter to take my picture during an interview. Both got interested in Yoga and admitted they badly needed it because, as they said in their own words, "anyone who works in the offices of a newspaper has an ulcer or suffers from tension."

If you want to see how the ribs expand during inhalation and how they contract during exhalation, watch yourself in the mirror. Of course, the chest should then remain uncovered. You will also experience the joy of "discovering your lungs," and of knowing that you can consciously take a deep breath and direct it to any part of the body you desire.

Exercises for the Neck and Eyes

Now we are going to start the exercises for the neck and eyes that will help do away with eyestrain, tension and stiffness of the neck. You can do them whenever you please—at the beginning of the lesson, at the end, or at any other time.

Many of my students practice these exercises while taking a bath, listening to the radio, or at intervals while at work, whether at a computer or doing housework. One of my friends does them in the car while waiting for his wife to finish shopping; another, while the commercials are on, when watching TV. It all depends on how much time one has to spare.

Before starting these exercises, see for yourself how flexible your neck is; then decide whether or not it needs to be exercised.

Just drop your head forward, then rotate it several times. If the rolling goes smoothly without any grinding or crackling noises you have nothing to worry about; if it doesn't, it will be best then to try the neck exercises.

Usually the trouble begins when the joints, or rather their linings, are inadequately lubricated and begin to stiffen from accumulation of calcium deposits—a sign of old age regardless of how old you are. As one new student remarked once after finishing the exercises, "It sounds as if I were eating gravel." This crunching sound is certainly a warning of impending trouble—unnecessary trouble, too, as one can preserve one's elasticity, health, and youthful appearance by spending a few minutes a day doing the right type of exercise.

NECK EXCERCISES

Sit on the floor with your legs crossed and keep the hands on the knees. If you prefer to sit on a chair, choose a hard one, otherwise you will find it difficult to keep your back straight, which is essential.

Relax the whole body. You should be conscious of it and only move it from the neck up; the rest should remain motionless and as unperturbed as if you were sitting under water up to the neck.

1) Now close your eyes and inhale; effortlessly and gently let your head drop forward while you exhale. Next, while you inhale let it drop backward. Repeat this exercise four times at the beginning. Later on you can increase the number to six or more. When dropping the head backward keep your facial muscles relaxed and your lips slightly parted.

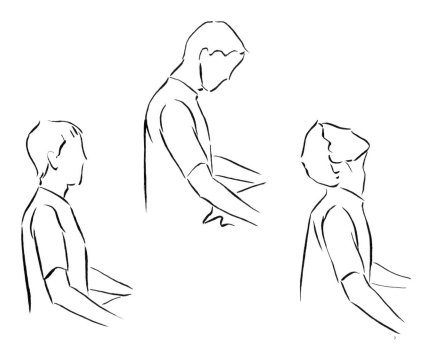

2) In the next exercise, first inhale and, while turning your head to the right, begin to exhale; return to normal position while inhaling. Next, turn your head completely to the left while exhaling, and once again return it to normal position while inhaling. Repeat four times. Turning the head to both sides contracts the muscles; returning to normal position relaxes them. Remember to breathe through your nose.

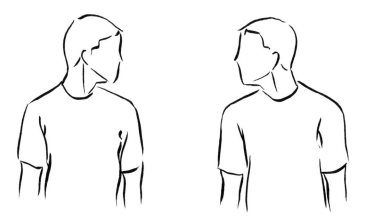

3) In the third exercise, first inhale, and then bend your head to the right, as if someone were pulling your right ear toward the right shoulder, while exhaling. Straighten the head once again while inhaling. Bend it to the left again while exhaling, and straighten again while inhaling. Repeat four times. When bending the head to the side, be sure not to lift the shoulder, tense it or tilt the head—you should move it only from its upright position to an almost horizontal one, otherwise there will be very little pull in the neck. You should feel this pull strongly in the left side of the neck when the head is bent to the right, and in the right side when the head is bent to the left.

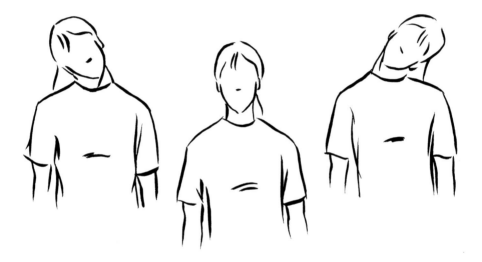

4) The next exercise resembles a turtle's neck movements, for you should literally "stick your neck out" as far as you can, and then draw it in again. In doing so, you will make a gliding movement forward with your chin, as if trying to reach out with it and thus lengthen the neck. Here you should feel the pull in the back of your neck on both sides, between the ears as well as in the middle. Repeat this exercise four times.

5) In the last exercise, do the same movement that you did to test the elasticity of your neck. Drop your head forward and feel it grow limp and heavy; then let it roll slowly clockwise several times; repeat counterclockwise the same number of times. Do not stiffen your back or

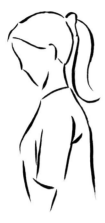 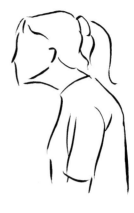

shoulders, but let the head hang relaxed, like that of a sleeping baby or someone who has had too many drinks. Remember to inhale when the head goes back and to exhale when it comes forward.

At the end of the last exercise, pat the neck and under the chin with the back of both hands. To pat the back of the neck, use your palms and fingertips.

The daily practice of these exercises will loosen up the tension in your neck muscles and keep them relaxed and supple. It will also control any tendency to a double chin and help to improve your eyesight. Vision gets better and clearer as the ophthalmic or eye nerves receive a richer supply of blood.

EYE EXERCISES

Remain in the same position as before. Make sure you are seated correctly. Is your spine straight? Hands on knees? Body relaxed? Head erect? This is how you should always remain while doing the eye exercises. The whole body must be motionless; nothing must move except the eyes.

Now raise your eyes and find a small point that you can see clearly, without frowning, without becoming tense and, of course, without moving your head. While doing this exercise look at this point each time you raise your eyes.

Next, lower your eyes to find a small point on the floor that you can see clearly when glancing down. Look at it each time you lower your eyes. Breathing should be normal—that is, you don't have to deep breathe.

TECHNIQUE:
1) a. Raise the eyes to look at the chosen high point.
    b. Lower the eyes to look at the chosen low point.
    c. Repeat four times. Close the eyes and rest a moment.

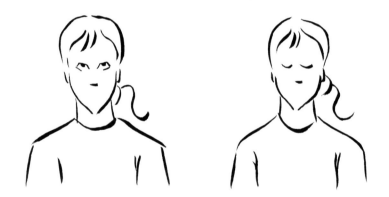

2) Now look for two other points, one to your left and one to your right, at eye level. You may also raise a finger on each side, or two pencils as guides and adjust them so that you can see them clearly when moving the eyes to the right and to the left, but without straining.

Keeping the fingers at eye level, and moving only the eyes, look to the right at your chosen point, then to the left. Repeat four times. Blink several times, then close your eyes and rest.

3) Next choose a point you can see from the right corner of your eyes when you raise them, and another that you can see from the left corner of your eyes when you lower them, half closing the lids. Remember to retain your original posture—spine erect, hands on knees, head straight and motionless.

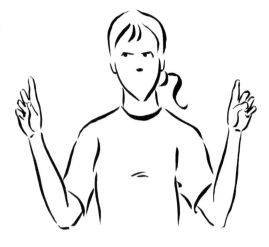

Look at your chosen point in the right corner up, then to the one in the left corner down. Repeat four times. Blink several times. Close the eyes and rest.

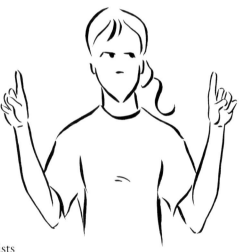

4) Next is an exercise which should not be done until three or four days after you have begun the course. It consists of slowly rolling the eyes first clockwise, then counterclockwise as follows: Lower your eyes and look at the floor, then slowly move the eyes to the left, higher and higher until you see the ceiling. Now continue circling to the right, lower and lower down, until you see the floor again. Do this slowly, making a full vision circle. Blink, close your eyes and rest. Then repeat the same movement counterclockwise.

5) Next comes a changing-vision exercise. While doing it you alternately shift your vision from close to distant points several times.

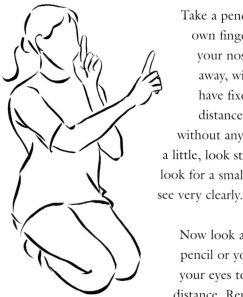

Take a pencil, for example, or use your own finger and put it on the tip of your nose. Then start moving it away, without raising it, until you have fixed it at the closest possible distance where you can see it clearly without any blur. Then raise your eyes a little, look straight into the distance and look for a small point that you can also see very clearly.

Now look at the closer point—the pencil or your fingertip—then shift your eyes to the farther point in the distance. Repeat several times, blink, close your eyes and squeeze. Then release.

6) And now for the palming which is most important for preserving the eyesight. Palming has a beneficial and relaxing effect on your nervous system.

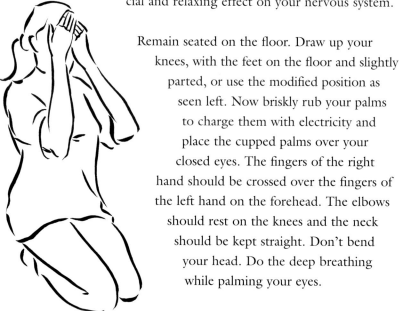

Remain seated on the floor. Draw up your knees, with the feet on the floor and slightly parted, or use the modified position as seen left. Now briskly rub your palms to charge them with electricity and place the cupped palms over your closed eyes. The fingers of the right hand should be crossed over the fingers of the left hand on the forehead. The elbows should rest on the knees and the neck should be kept straight. Don't bend your head. Do the deep breathing while palming your eyes.

If you are going to do the palming for
longer than a few minutes, it is better
to sit down at a table, place some
books or pillows in front of you to
support your elbows, so that
you can keep the neck straight,
and place the cupped palms of
your hands on your eyes as
explained before. If you are going
to do a short exercise, you can
do deep breathing for half a
minute or so at first, and gradually increase
it every week.

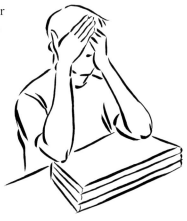

I met a blind woman, who came very early one Monday morning to
one of the Foundation centers in Buenos Aires. She had heard me on
the radio the day before while I was being interviewed, and felt such a
great surge of hope and trust that Yoga would help her regain her eyesight that she began to do the exercises she was told to. Thanks to her
perseverance, the practice of the Asanas, the meditation and to a great
deal of faith and hope on her part, she was able to partially regain her
lost vision.

Yoga Postures

*Of all creatures, the human being has the least sense for
management of his body.*

—EHRENFRIED E. PFEIFFER, M.D., Ph.D

You are now ready to start learning the Yoga postures. Naturally we
shall begin with the simplest ones; then, as your joints and muscles
become more nimble and flexible, we will go on to those that are

more difficult to do. Please don't allow yourself to be frightened away or easily discouraged. Remember these are not calisthenics, that you are not competing against yourself or anyone else, and that the exercises must not be forced. Feel happy if you make slow progress. You will be amazed to discover how much your body will be able to do in a short time.

ROCKING

Let us begin with the strengthening Rocking exercise. This exercise helps overcome the drowsiness and stiffness that one so often feels on waking up in the morning. As you do the Rocking exercise, you will also feel an agreeable, invigorating sensation because of the healthy massage your vertebrae are receiving. This exercise will make your spine more flexible and keep it in a supple and youthful condition. The yogis say that you can dodge old age as long as your spine remains elastic and strong. Rocking will also help you to sleep better and more

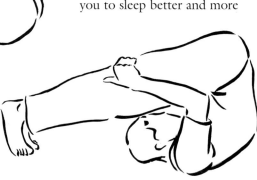

soundly. I remember the effect it had on one of my students, an officer in the British army, who had been suffering from insomnia for a long time. About a week after he started studying with me, he burst into the class triumphantly announcing that he had slept through the night without any pills. He has probably been sleeping like a baby ever since.

Rocking is actually a very simple exercise, and in a few days you will be able to do it without any kind of difficulty, whatever your age, the stiffness in your joints and even your weight.

TECHNIQUE: Sit down at the end of the exercise mat to make sure your back does not suffer the floor's hardness. Draw up your knees, and bend your head down, keeping your chin tucked in against your sternum and rounding your spine. Take hold of your legs with your hands under your knees. You can join your hands or not, whichever is easiest in the beginning.

Now, keeping your spine rounded, swing back and forth, back and forth, in quick successive movements imitating the swinging motions of a rocking chair. Don't straighten your spine as you rock backward or you will find yourself lying flat on your back, unable to swing forward again. Don't try to do the rocking movement too slowly either, at least in the beginning. Just imagine you are a rocking chair in motion, and enjoy the fun of it.

Here is another helpful hint: straighten the knees just as you swing backwards and then immediately bend them again as you swing forward. Don't pause after you have swung back, but continue the to-and-fro movement. Otherwise, you may get "stuck" and stop.

You may feel a little clumsy and awkward the first day, and you may even be afraid of losing your balance and falling down. Remember you are already on the floor, so this can hardly happen. In a few days, when you grow used to rocking, you will probably enjoy this exercise as much as I do, and you will notice its strengthening and invigorating effects. Again, remember to keep your spine rounded and the head bent forward all the time, otherwise you will bump it against the floor when you swing backward and never again want to do this exercise, which, on the other hand, I am sure will become your favorite among all others.

On the second and third days, you can try to combine the Rocking exercise with deep breathing. Inhale while rocking backward and exhale while returning forward. Be sure not to have any zippers, buttons, hoods or buckles in the way or you may be in for an unpleasant sensation when rocking backward.

TIME: Do this exercise four to six times, then lie down to relax until your breath returns to normal again; finally take a few deep breaths while still lying on the floor.

BENEFITS: The Rocking exercise stimulates the flow of nervous energy through the spinal cord and establishes a better connection between the central nervous system and the rest of the body.

RAISED-LEGS POSTURE
(Uddhita Padasana)

Your next exercise will be the Raised-Legs Posture, Udhitta Padasana in Sanskrit. Its technique is not difficult to grasp, but it may take a little time before you are able to execute it properly.

TECHNIQUE: Lie down on your back, hands along your sides with palms down on the floor and knees and legs together. Inhale a deep breath while raising the right leg—keeping straight and with the foot's sole toward the ceiling—until it is at a right angle to your body. Hold your breath without making any effort, and stay in this position without bending the knee, keeping the other leg flat on the floor. Then start exhaling while you slowly bring down the right leg again.

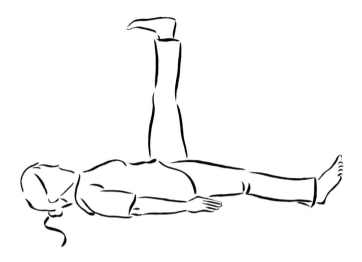

Repeat the same exercise with the left leg and then
with both legs at the same time. Now take a rest.

TIME: Hold this posture three seconds, gradually
increasing it to ten seconds. At the beginning do the
exercise only once or twice. After a few days you
can try raising and lowering
both legs together four or
five times without stopping.
If you want to hold the posture for a longer period of
time, practice regular breathing.

BENEFITS: This posture gives the
abdomen an internal vibrating massage, thereby strengthening the
muscles and reducing the fatty tissue. It is a good exercise for people
who have a flabby abdomen. It is also good for people with varicose
veins, because it improves blood flow.

You may find it difficult at the beginning to lower both legs slowly,
especially as they come closer to the floor. However, you will improve

before the week is over. Your abdominal muscles will probably feel a little sore the day after you start, as this exercise gives them a strong massage, but this will only be temporary.

CAUTION: This posture should not be done by women during the first days of menstruation, or by anyone with a weak heart or suffering from high blood pressure. For people with serious lumbar problems, it is best to raise and lower legs flexed.

HEAD-TO-KNEE POSTURE
(Janushirshasana)

Next we shall do the Head-to-Knee Posture, called Janushirshasana in Sanskrit—from Janu meaning knee, Shirsh meaning head, and Asana meaning posture.

TECHNIQUE: Sit up straight with both legs stretched out and toes pointing toward the ceiling. Then bend the left leg and place the sole of the left foot against the right thigh, as close as you can to the genital area.

Inhale deeply, slightly stretch the upper part of the body by raising the arms; draw in the stomach, then exhale slowly, while bending forward from the waist to get hold of your right foot with both hands. Your forehead should touch the right knee. Hold your breath for a few seconds. Then go back to the original position while you inhale and come up with your head between your arms.

TIME: Remain in this posture for five seconds and gradually increase the time to ten seconds. Repeat once or twice, then reverse legs and try to bring the forehead to the left knee. After this, lie down and relax. Take a few deep breaths before sitting up again. When you reach the point where you are able to keep this posture for a longer period than you can hold your breath, simply resume normal breathing, while you take advantage of each exhalation to relax and come closer to the knee.

BENEFITS: The Head-to-Knee Posture is a helpful exercise in more than one way. It is good for preventing or relieving indigestion, constipation, and troubles arising from an enlarged spleen. It tones up slow bowels, strengthens the legs and adds to your energy and vitality.

In the beginning you will probably find it difficult to reach your outstretched foot with your hands. You may even begin to wonder whether your arms are not too short. The fault, however, is usually not with the arms, but with the abdomen that has grown too large or with the spine that has lost its flexibility. The moment you become suppler, you will find no difficulty in reaching your feet.

Meanwhile, simply get hold of your calves, ankles, or toes and grasp them firmly while trying to bring your head closer to the knee, even if it does take some time before you are actually able to reach the

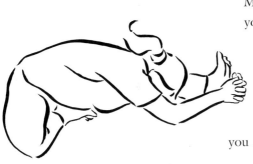

knee with your forehead. You should not feel discouraged by your lack of immediate success. I too had some difficulty when I first started practicing this posture, and never thought I would be able to accomplish this feat. The important thing if you want positive results is to keep practicing daily.

You may find it easier to do this exercise with the aid of a strap or belt, as shown in the picture. As you bend forward, shorten the strap, letting your hands come closer and closer to your foot. You will be surprised to find that in a comparatively short time you will be able to grasp your toes—something that seemed to be completely beyond your reach not so long ago.

After you have taken a short rest, sit up again in the same Head-to-Knee Pose to do the next exercise, which will eventually enable you to assume the Lotus Pose.

LOTUS POSE
(Padmasana)

In order to prepare yourself, place the sole of your right foot against the left thigh, and begin making a bouncing up and down movement with your right knee as though it were made of rubber, that is, the moment the knee touches the floor, up it bounces again. Do this bouncing in fast successive movements so that the leg resembles the wing of a flying bird. This exercise will stretch your stiff ligaments and muscles, making them more flexible and gradually allowing you to assume the Lotus Pose. First bounce the right knee, then do the same with the left.

There is a variation to this exercise, which is done as follows: place the right foot on the left thigh instead of placing it against the thigh; then start bouncing the right knee as shown in the picture.

If the bouncing knee easily touches the floor, then bend the left knee, take the left foot with both hands, slide it over the right crossed leg and place the foot on the right thigh. Now both legs are symmetrically crossed and you are sitting in the Lotus Pose.

The hands should be kept on the knees. You can also keep the palms open, with the thumb and second finger of each touching, forming a letter O.

It often happens that new students, who never thought they could do it, are able to assume this posture during their first lesson. But mostly, it takes some time before people are able to master the Lotus Pose. This is why you should keep on practicing the exercise of bouncing the knees daily, until eventually your knee does hit the floor. This will be a sign that your legs are sufficiently flexible for this posture.

Another variation for stretching the coccyx-femoral joint articulation is the "butterfly wing-flutter." Flex your two legs, bring the soles of your feet together taking the

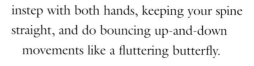

instep with both hands, keeping your spine straight, and do bouncing up-and-down movements like a fluttering butterfly.

The Lotus Pose, or Padmasana, is one of the basic Yoga postures. The others are the Headstand, the Shoulderstand, the Plough, the Cobra, the Twist and the Stretching Postures. There are also the Stomach Lift, the Yoga Mudra and the Reverse Pose. The last two are not called Asanas, or postures, but Mudras, which means gestures; and the Stomach Lift is called Uddyiana Bandha—Bandha meaning restraint or contraction.

For thousands of years, the Padmasana has been assumed in India not only by the rishis (wise men) and yogis, but by ordinary people as well. Because of its calming effect upon the mind and the nerves, it has become a classical pose for concentration and meditation. Many Indians, especially in the South, also sit in this pose when working, reading, writing or eating. It makes it easier to keep the spine erect, which as I have already said is a must in Yoga. In the West, the Lotus Posture is often called the Buddha Pose, because most paintings and sculptures of the Enlightened One represent him seated in the Lotus Posture, with the hands on the knees or on the upturned heels.

In India one often sees people in deep meditation sitting motionless in this posture for hours. It has no special therapeutic value except to keep the joints in flexible condition and hold the spine erect, both necessary for breathing practices. It also helps develop a good posture.

COBRA POSE
(Bhujanghasana)

The posture you are about to do next is called the Cobra Pose, or Bhujanghasana in Sanskrit. It belongs to the basic group of Yoga postures. You will find it easy to do, especially if your back is not too stiff and rigid. But even if your back is not too flexible, you will be able to do the Cobra, though not perfectly at first.

TECHNIQUE: Lie down on your stomach with your feet and knees together, stretched insteps, flexed elbows, and the palms of the hands placed on the floor at shoulder level. The arms should remain close to the body with the elbows facing the ceiling, the forehead on the floor.

Now while inhaling a deep breath, slowly raise the head, then the shoulders, the chest and the upper part of the body—the lower part of the body should remain flat on the floor. Hold your breath and keep arching the spine until you feel strong pressure in the lower part of the back. Do not straighten the arms; they must stay flexed. Remain in this posture for a few seconds. Then begin to exhale as you slowly lower the body until the forehead touches the floor. Repeat once more and relax.

When you bend the body backwards be sure not to do any violent movement, as you may damage a stiff muscle. Raise your body very gradually and slowly, like a cobra that hoists up or like a sphinx. After finishing the Cobra, and because of the effort put in, you should rest in the Child Posture (Pindasana): sitting on the heels with stretched insteps, bend for-ward until you touch your forehead to the floor; the arms go back and to the sides of the body, with the palms facing upwards.

TIME: Keep the pose for five seconds, gradually increasing to ten seconds. Do the exercises from two to seven times, adding one time every 14 days. If you feel you can hold the posture for a longer period of time, continue breathing regularly through your nose.

BENEFITS: The Cobra Posture affects the adrenal glands that are situated above each kidney, pumping a richer supply of blood into them. This posture is also beneficial for backache due to overwork or long hours of standing. It adjusts displacements in the spinal column and tones the sympathetic nerves. It is an especially good exercise for women suffering from ovarian and uterine problems. This posture is also practiced to increase body heat. People troubled with gas after meals will find the Cobra Posture to be very helpful.

CAUTION: Women going through their period should not practice this exercise; neither should people with high blood pressure, serious coronary problems, pain in the lumbar area or a herniated disk. In such cases, they may practice the half cobra, placing the palms of the hands, forearms and elbows on the floor. Those who have problems in the cervical area should not pull the head too far back.

SQUATTING POSE
(Utkasana)

Now get up to try the Squatting Pose, called Utkasana in Sanskrit, which requires no particular skill or special preparation. It is only when the knees have become too stiff that one will have difficulties practicing it.

In the Orient, especially in India, the common people often sit this way. You can see them squatting on sidewalks and beaches, in doorways and railway stations. Once, a rich Indian who owned a graphite factory

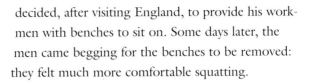

decided, after visiting England, to provide his work-men with benches to sit on. Some days later, the men came begging for the benches to be removed: they felt much more comfortable squatting.

TECHNIQUE:

FIRST VERSION: Stand with your legs open and your feet about a foot apart. Take a deep breath while rising on your tiptoes; then, while exhaling, start lowering your body until you are sitting on your heels. Slowly rise again to standing position, keeping your back straight the whole time.

SECOND VERSION: Proceed as above, but with-out raising your heels from the ground. Then sit in a squat so that your buttocks are almost touching the floor. Your body should be slightly bent forward and your thighs pressing against the abdomen.

There is a THIRD VER-SION which is much more difficult, as you must squat with your feet together and without rais-ing your heels off the ground.

Repeat any of the variations three or four times or do each one once. Then lie down to take a few deep breaths.

If your knees have lost their flexibility and you are unable to do the Squatting Pose, start by doing it holding on to a doorknob with both hands (open the door and grasp the knobs on both sides), or grasping the arms of a heavy chair or anything else that will hold your weight without toppling over, such as a piano, bed, sofa, or pillar. Gradually lower your body more and more, making little swinging movements. In a few days you will be able to squat better.

This posture helps restore flexibility to stiff and aching knees and to get relief from lumbago. It makes stair-climbing very easy and is a great exercise for skiers and hikers.

However, these are not the main reasons for teaching you this exercise: the main purpose is that the Squatting Pose contributes to better intestinal elimination. This is the posture designed by nature itself for evacuation of waste matter, because the spine is slightly bent forward and the thighs are pressed against the abdomen. The use of high-seat toilets in the West is probably one of the main reasons for the increasing number of sufferers from poor elimination and constipation. And these ailments in turn are directly or indirectly the cause of a host of other troubles and diseases.

There is but one disease, according to the once world-famous surgeon Sir W. A. Lane: insufficient and inadequate drainage of toxic waste materials. Unless they are disposed of, they continue poisoning the system and begin to slowly undermine the health until they finally destroy it.

A governess of the children of one of my friends used to make the little ones practice the Squatting Pose for when they went to the bathroom. She herself had never had any elimination problem in France, where she had been brought up, because they used floor-level toilets without a seat.

Also in Japan and in India the toilets are at floor level, except, naturally, those in the houses built for foreigners.

This is not an aesthetic matter for discussion; nevertheless, it is one of huge importance for our well-being and should not be lightly dismissed or made fun of.

The Squat is your last posture for today. You should not overtire yourself, especially since this is your first lesson.

Breathing Exercises

You will now learn two breathing exercises. The first is very beneficial for people suffering from asthma. The second is especially suitable for those who suffer sacroiliac troubles.

FIRST BREATHING EXERCISE

Lie down flat on your back and place your feet on the wall as high as you can; extend your arms out above your head keeping the elbows straight. Now do deep breathing while remaining in this position. Start with four deep breaths, then gradually increase the number. You may practice this exercise even lying on a bed. Incidentally, people suffering from asthma will benefit greatly from this breathing exercise.

SECOND BREATHING EXERCISE

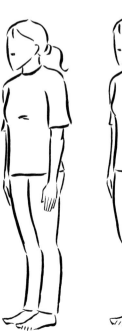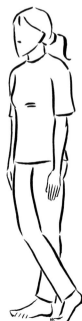

Stand straight, feet together, hands at your sides, keeping the spine very straight. Cross the right foot over the left one, keeping the toes on the floor, but the heel off, and the back part of the right knee on top of the left knee. Do not straighten your legs or move your body to the left—it is extremely important that the spine remain centered.

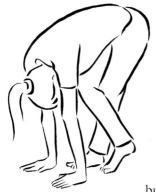

Now take a deep breath. Then exhale while you bend forward until you touch the floor with your fingertips or come as near to touching it as you can manage. Return to standing position and do a deep breath.

Do this exercise three times, then reverse the legs and feet and repeat. When you bend forward, be sure not to move your buttocks or shoulders. Only the spine, starting from the waistline up, should do the bending.

If done correctly, this exercise removes the "morning" backaches. People suffering from sacroiliac troubles should do this exercise twice a day to feel relief.

Relaxation
(Savasana)

Your lesson for today is over and you will finish it with a period of complete rest and relaxation.

First, stand up straight and relax your hands by shaking them a bit to loosen them up, as if trying to shake water drops from your fingers. Do the same with your right foot and then with the left one. Now stretch your arms above your head as if trying to reach for the sun with your hands, rise on tiptoe and stretch as high as you can.

Next, you must slowly let your body become limp until it feels completely heavy; pretend you are a lotus flower that is drooping and folding its long stem and slowly sink to the floor. Lie down and close your eyes. This lifeless pose is called Savasana in Sanskrit, and, even if it appears to be very easy, requires practice.

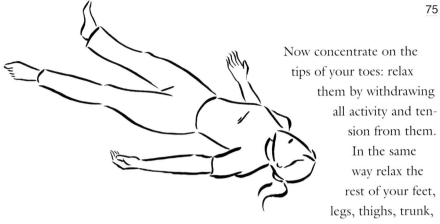

Now concentrate on the tips of your toes: relax them by withdrawing all activity and tension from them. In the same way relax the rest of your feet, legs, thighs, trunk, and back. Let the feeling of relaxation and laziness slowly overtake your whole body. Relax your shoulders, arms, and fingers. Drop your chin and let the lower jaw sag to relax the muscles of the face. Now try feeling so heavy you are sinking into the floor, while remaining fully relaxed and completely at ease.

Lie like this, motionless, for a while. Then take a few deep breaths and try to visualize a cloud—a soft white cloud drifting in the sky. Hold this image for some time, then dismiss it. Now imagine that you are this cloud. You feel

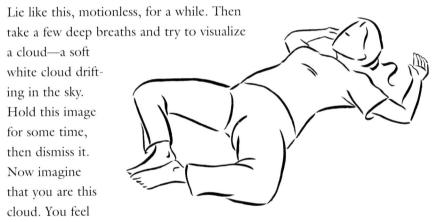

light, completely relaxed, floating in the sky, passing another cloud, gently gliding over a green valley, a field, a forest, above a small lake in which you see yourself reflected. How pleasant to feel so airy, so free and happy! You are but a cloud in the vast blue sky.

Now try to dismiss all thoughts from your mind and make it completely blank, leaving it hollow and thoughtless, as if you were sinking into oblivion, into nothingness, fully relaxed, peaceful, calm, and quiet.

Stay like this as long as you wish. Then begin slowly, very slowly, to stretch your body. First stretch your arms above your head, yawning deeply. Stretch your hands, fingers, shoulders, spine, and legs. Roll over on your right side and arch your back. Roll to the left side, arching once again. Lie again on your back. After a while, start to sit slowly, always yawning and stretching, if you need it.

You may now get up and go about your business. But in our classes we always finish the lesson with a period of meditation in which everyone joins, including those who have taken up Yoga merely to get rid of some extra weight, eliminate premature wrinkles or get over constipation, tension, insomnia or other similar causes of distress.

We simply sit down in the Lotus Pose or else cross-legged, close our eyes and take a few deep breaths. Then we stay very still, trying to direct our thoughts to the Infinite Light that is Truth, Love, God, or whatever you wish to call the superior force, beyond form, beyond our understanding. We try to realize that It is everywhere, both outside us and within us; that we, as human beings, are the carriers of the Divine Light here on Earth that dwells in our hearts; that our bodies are the Temple of the Divine Light and we should try for this Light to shine through our eyes, speak through our words and express itself in our deeds.

Then we send a thought of peace and love to all those around us, to our family, to our friends, to the people we love, to those we do not love, to all living beings on this Earth and beyond. At the end, we say aloud:

Let me go
from the unreal to the Real,
from the darkness to the Light
from death to Immortality
OM
Shanti, shanti, shanti

In our classes at the Indra Devi Foundation centers in Buenos Aires, we intone this old Vedic chant, called the Asato Maa:

Asato maa sad gamaya
Tamaso maa jyotir gamaya
Mrtyor maa 'mrtam gamaya
Om shanti shanti shanti

OM is the sacred sound of the Hindus, and shanti means peace in Sanskrit.

You may also sing any other prayer with whatever wording you choose: this is up to you. But I suggest that at least once a day you remind yourself that you are of divine origin and that you are on this Earth to bring love, peace, and goodness to all living creatures.

General Rules and Recommendations

Let us now recapitulate your first lesson item by item.

While still in bed you did the alternate stretching of the legs.

Then you learned to do deep breathing.

Next, you did the neck and the eye exercises.

Then came the Rocking exercise, the Raised-Legs Posture, the Head-to-Knee Posture, the preparatory exercise of knee bouncing for the Lotus Pose, the Cobra, the Squatting Posture, the two breathing exercises, and, finally, the relaxation.

If you have never done any of these exercises or have not been doing them for a long time, it is advisable the first day to start only with the breathing, the neck and eye exercises, one or two postures, and the relaxation. Then, gradually, add the remaining postures day by day, trying not to overexert yourself.

Now let us go over some general rules and suggestions regarding the exercises and hygiene.

1) Always do the exercises on an empty stomach; allow three hours after meals; one and a half to two hours after breakfast or a light snack. Never exercise when the bladder is full. Never eat immediately after the exercises, but wait for about half an hour before taking a meal. This is especially important if you have been doing strenuous exercises for an hour or so.

2) Exercise in a well-ventilated room or out in the open air.

3) Do not exercise for more than fifteen to twenty minutes during the first few days.

4) Rest frequently between exercises.

5) After the first three weeks, the actual exercise time should not exceed an hour.

6) Don't wear tight clothes while doing the exercises.

7) Yoga postures are always accompanied by deep breathing, which is done with the mouth closed.

8) After a long illness, resume the exercises slowly. For the first few days do only the breathing, the relaxation and the neck and eye exercises.

9) The same rule holds for women during the days of their period.

10) Women who are more than three months pregnant should refrain from the more strenuous exercises.

11) Don't feel concerned if the exercises produce a sense of fatigue during the first days; this tired feeling will soon disappear. It is usually caused by toxin excess. I suggest you try resting and not try to fight off this fatigue.

12) Take good care of your teeth. Rinse your mouth after every meal; cleanse your tongue as well.

13) Internal cleanliness is an important requirement for maintaining good health. Keep your body free of toxins by drinking a lot of water between meals, but don't drink water during meals and never drink ice water.

14) It is advisable to take an enema once in a while, even if you are not constipated. In order to get rid of toxic waste matter, I recommend taking an enema in the morning (or evening) before you begin this home course. One of the most effective cleansers for this purpose is a honey or a coffee enema. However, it is best to consult a doctor about its use in each case.

Prepare the honey enema in the following way: Dissolve three tablespoons of honey in a quart of tepid water at room temperature; hold the enema from ten to fifteen minutes.

The coffee enema is made as follows: Add three tablespoons of ground coffee to a quart of boiling water. Do not use instant coffee. Let it boil three minutes; then simmer another twelve minutes. Strain it. Cool to room temperature. Take the enema and hold it for ten to fifteen minutes.

This may sound strange to you, but when coffee is introduced through the colon, it does not react on the nervous system; instead, it stimulates the solar plexus and lever secretions by affecting the adrenal glands and the gall bladder. It also activates the mucous membrane of the colon and thus helps to eliminate the accumulated toxins. A coffee enema would therefore also contribute to arrest the beginning of a cold or to relieve a toxic headache. However, it is best not to take a coffee enema late in the evening, to avoid being kept awake at night.

15) Do not sleep with light in your room.

16) Sleep in a well-ventilated room, with windows open, if possible.

17) Do not sleep with plants or flowers in your bedroom because they give off carbon dioxide at night, whereas during the day they release oxygen.

18) Sleep with the feet toward the Equator, and the head toward the Pole, that is, parallel to, and not across the magnetic-force lines of the earth.

19) Most people get their best sleep before midnight, so don't keep late hours.

20) Sleep with as little clothing as possible; it is better yet not to have anything on the body.

21) It is always advisable to check your heart, lungs and blood pressure before starting your Yoga instruction.

At the end of our next lesson, we will have a lengthy discussion on the issues regarding food regimes. Meanwhile, it is best for you to cut down on fried, fatty and heavy foods, as well as on liquor. Finally, even though its ill effects are greatly diminished by deep breathing, I advise you to stop smoking.

Discussion: On the Effects of Breathing

In our classes we often hold discussions at the end of the lesson, on various subjects directly or indirectly related to Yoga.

As you already know, Yoga is both a science and an art of living, and, therefore, affects innumerable facets of our daily life, from cleansing the skin to cleansing the mind, from a broken ligament to a sad heart, from transcendent issues regarding marriage to overweight problems and delinquency troubles. There are actually very few matters on which Yoga has nothing to say. I consider it appropriate to also address some of these issues in this book after each one of our lessons because they might be of interest and help to the reader.

We will begin with breathing—the essence not only of all Yoga practices but of all life. Breathing is the most important of all our functions, for without breathing we would not be able to live more than a few minutes. However, most people don't know much about the effects that breathing has on our body and mind; and still less about the role it plays in bringing forth the spirit within us.

Our blood and entire organism is composed of millions and millions of tiny cells that feed on the oxygen we carry in our blood stream by virtue of our breathing.

To have a clear understanding of the major role breathing plays in sustaining life, we have only to remember that not a single tissue cell can be built without red blood, and in turn, not a single red blood cell can be built without oxygen.

Try comparing a cell to a balloon: Inflated with air, it is firm and tense, because of which it can fly up into the skies; but if it develops a leak, it soon loses all its tone, begins to shrivel, and finally falls to the ground.

The same is true of each cell in our body. Unless provided with sufficient oxygen it becomes depleted, tired and lifeless. As a result the whole body begins to lose its youthfulness and vitality.

The life and functions of each cell are sustained by oxygen, which dominates the activities of the entire body. Oxygen is a vital factor in the composition of minerals, the maintenance of normal electrical potentials, and it carries out a main role in illnesses and in the disposal of waste material.

We ourselves are rarely completely aware of all these complex processes going on in our bodies day and night, year in and year out. However, we do know that without oxygen they would all come to a standstill. It is therefore our duty to assist the body in this unending task, and we can do this by learning how to expand our breathing capacity.

Oxygen is also essential to the proper function of each of our internal organs; the most demanding of which is our brain, to the point of requiring three times the amount of oxygen used by all the rest of the body.

In the United States there are more than five million mentally retarded children. According to Dr. Philip Rice, who dedicated his life to the rehabilitation of so-called problem children, many of these unfortunate youngsters are the victims of a lack of oxygen in their brains and their condition may greatly improve by putting them through a program of correct breathing exercises. He also feels that these same exercises would be of equal benefit in many cases of juvenile delinquency.

In his excellent book *Building for Mental and Physical Health,* Dr. Philip Rice states that the I.Q. of a child can be increased by enlarging the intake of oxygen his organism absorbs through correct deep breathing. However, he strongly condemns the wrong kind of "deep breathing" (in which the upper part of the chest is raised) qualifying it as a "thoroughly pernicious method." Incidentally, this is exactly the kind of breathing that is usually taught in schools, gyms and health clubs.

An inadequate supply of oxygen gradually impairs the function of the organs, speeds up the aging process and results in weakness and ill health of the body and mind. A person who is used to deep breathing need not worry—he or she can protect himself/herself against all of these troubles. But as it happens, civilized man is a shallow breather, who uses only one third of his lung capacity while rarely, if ever, using the rest.

How can a man then expect to think, to create, to work and live in full measure if he never uses more than one-third of his breathing capacity? He cannot expect to receive adequate nourishment for his cell functions, no matter how well and how much he feeds himself with his mouth, because the various processes of nutrition demand oxygen for the proper molecular exchange between the nutritive elements and the tissues. When you breathe properly, the energy is fully released, and it can produce a larger amount of enzymes to preserve life.

Dr. Max Jacobson of New York, who was the first to isolate enzymes and reduce them to their pure form, believes that in order to maintain a healthy cell-life and to foster cell renewal and survival, proper oxygen metabolism is crucial and essential.

Getting the most out of our bodies by supplying it with oxygen is like getting a nut out of a shell with the help of a nutcracker. Therefore, if you want to have a good digestion, do not neglect deep breathing, which provides the organism with additional oxygen. The same advice holds for smokers. Talking to them about the possible dangers of excessive smoking is useless. They are probably more familiar than I am with all the literature linking cigarette consumption to cancer of the throat and lungs. Their hoarse coughing alone should be a warning signal that something is wrong in their bodies. If they would at least do five or ten deep breathings after each cigarette, they would ventilate their otherwise chronically congested and clogged lungs.

The yogis, who have known for several thousand years about the incredible power of breathing, have successfully worked out an unsurpassed technique of utilizing this power for man's benefit. Deep breathing, as taught by them, can work wonders on tired, sick, and aging bodies as well as on restless, tense, and fearful minds.

Tension, insomnia, indigestion, constipation, nervous headaches, heart conditions, as well as mental disorders—including delinquency—are often the result of insufficient oxygen intake. Unfortunately, most authorities, whether at home, in schools, hospitals, prisons or other similar institutions, have not yet fully recognized the importance of deep breathing.

Even doctors rarely, as it seems, acknowledge the degree to which the health and well-being of their patients depends on their breathing habits, although they do hurry to take oxygen tanks to the sick person's bedside in case of an emergency, as when a person suffers a stroke.

Interesting observations on the results of oxygen starvation have been made by the English Frank Totney, who in his small book *Oxygen, Master of Cancer,* insists that cancer is caused by oxygen deficiency in the cells, which rapidly start to multiply in order to find what they need. I am in no position to judge whether he is right or wrong, but I do know that his ideas for cancer prevention very closely resemble the Yoga principles of breathing, diet, exercising and hygiene. Just like yogis, he believes in the need to keep the body internally clean by means of deep breathing, drinking more water (a glass for every four-teen pounds of body weight each day), eating plenty of fresh fruit, salads and vegetables, and the purification of the colon by taking enemas about twice a month or so. In short, his idea is to rid the system of the accumulated poisons that are the direct cause of most of our ailments.

As man begins to get older, his life forces begin to slacken and he comes closer to receiving the mineralizing earth forces. The cells of his body become less elastic, losing their ability to absorb oxygen like they did before. Hence the body begins to shrivel or grow fatter, due to excess fatty tissue, and to stiffen, because the organism is less capable of coping with all its functions and becomes exposed to a greater number of troubles.

A sufficient oxygen intake is absolutely necessary in order to prevent the physical and mental deterioration and the kind of old age most people are afraid of—an old age that is reckoned not so much by the number of years one has lived as by the decline and weakening of the body's functions and of its mental faculties. But as long as the human being does not know how to master his breathing, he will never become the master of his body and his mind, remaining their slave forever. Even the most common cold, for example, can turn an otherwise assertive, dynamic and enterprising person into a miserable one. I assure the reader that if we know how to breathe correctly, we can literally breathe away most of the illnesses, tension, fatigue and other troubles we are prone to, from lack of self-confidence to lack of confidence in God.

As I have already said, centuries ago yogis worked out the most complete and elaborate science or art of breathing ever known to man. Thanks to this system, they have managed to develop astonishing and seemingly supernatural faculties and powers, over and above their ability to keep their bodies young, strong and free of disease.

But even an ordinary man, not only a yogi, can gain a certain amount of control over his body and his mind by means of deep rhythmic breathing.

Breathing, incidentally, is our only direct contact with the outer world, as everything else comes to us as impressions through the senses. Since breath is of cosmic nature we can, by using it consciously, establish a connection between Earth and Cosmos within our own body.

All this does not happen overnight, of course. Steady and diligent work is required in order to achieve such results. Most Yoga practices, especially the advanced ones, are based on the mastery of the different breathing techniques. However, the majority of them are not well suited to Occidental man, and it is therefore best not to go into them in order to prevent possible dangers or even disasters.

Once, a couple from Seattle came to see me in Los Angeles because they had gotten into trouble by attempting Pranayama. Here is a direct quote from their letter, which tells its own story:

"We found a young Hindu, a university student, from whom we took five lessons. We were getting along splendidly until we started practicing Pranayama under his direction. Since then we have both felt miserable. In your book, *Forever Young, Forever Healthy,* you have rightly warned against practicing Pranayama."

This, I believe, should serve as an urgent warning to others.

The mastery of the advanced stages of Yoga requires long years of special preparation and training under conditions difficult to achieve within the limitations of the present-day Occidental way of life. Therefore, we should limit our attention to the practice of deep breathing, and especially rhythmic breathing, as this too increases the circulation and the flow of that mysterious life-energy that in Sanskrit is called Prana, meaning Breath, Absolute Energy. However, we shall discuss this subject later on, at the end of the Fourth Lesson.

Meanwhile, we will explain the importance of nutrition in our next lesson, and give you an idea of how to ward off the aging of the body's organism and preserve its youthfulness by learning to select the right kinds of foods.

Lesson Two • Second Week

*Physical control is merely a preparation for
mental control; only when the mind calms down does
the process of becoming one with the Reality begin.*

A week has now gone by since you started practicing Yoga exercises,
and you may have already noticed their effect, provided, of course,
that you have been doing them regularly. Let us check and see
whether you can detect any results so far.

Are you sleeping better or falling asleep more quickly? Has your evacuation improved? Do you feel more relaxed and experience a greater
sense of lightness? Are your personal problems a little less nagging
than they used to be?

On the other hand, your habitual aches and pains may have increased,
your limbs grown stiffer, your body more bloated. Perhaps you feel
sleepy and drowsy all day long. If this happens to be the case, please
do not get alarmed. In certain rather rare instances students of Yoga
do experience discomfort in the beginning, and this is the reason why
I always insist in making it a point to warn my own pupils that during
the first few weeks of exercises they may indeed feel worse. But this is
nothing to worry about.

Some people become worse before they start getting better. The poisons stirred up by exercise are felt in a more acute way, especially if the organism is in a very toxic state. It is like shaking a glass of water with sand settled in the bottom—the water gets muddy before it can be strained and the sand eliminated.

So don't feel discouraged should this be happening to you, but give your system a chance to go through the cleansing process. You will feel like a new person afterwards. I remember one of my new students actually complaining in class about the pain she felt because of the exercises. She didn't give up, however, and as a result she is now free of arthritis, asthma, and sinus problems, all of which had been plaguing her.

My own personal experience with Yoga was equally unpleasant. You may recollect that in the autobiographical notes in my previous book I mentioned how I swelled up instead of slimming down, until I could hardly get into my clothes, in spite of eating very little. Of course, that was a time I was not yet wearing saris exclusively, as I do now.

As suggested in the general rules in the first lesson, you should help the body get through the cleansing process faster by drinking plenty of water as well as taking a daily enema for about a week.

As for performing the Asanas, I suggest again that at this point you re-read all instructions carefully and check whether you are doing the exercises properly or whether you have interpreted them in your own way and are improvising without being aware of it.

Do not forget to deep breathe with every posture and do not hurry any of the exercises—do them SLOWLY! Avoid being like that old lady I once knew who allotted herself fifteen minutes every morning for her exercises, rushed through them at top speed, immensely pleased to have accomplished so much in so short a time, and then complained of being out of breath. When corrected and slowed down, she was amazed at how relaxed she felt after each session, and how strong she felt because of the Yoga postures and exercises.

Before beginning with our second lesson, let us first go over your exercise schedule. You must have decidedly worked one out by now and have come to realize which is the best time of day for your Asanas—whether morning, noon, or evening. As a matter of fact, it is also permissible to work out a divided schedule—to do, for example, one set of exercises in the morning and the rest at night. I do recommend, however, that as soon as you get out of bed you always begin your day with Rocking.

Once you finish the Rocking, go over the new postures given for the current week, and then continue with those exercises from the previous week that you personally need most. For instance, if you have sacroiliac trouble, don't fail to do the breathing exercise with the crossed-over foot. If constipated, practice the Head-to-Knee Posture or the Squatting Posture, and also the Yoga Mudra, which you will learn today. If you are troubled by a sore throat or bad tonsils, do not omit the Lion Posture, which is given in Lesson Three. For the rest, you can either choose those exercises you like best or do a series of them alternately, depending on the amount of time you have at your disposal. But under no circumstances should you skip the basic Asanas.

Now let us begin with the actual lesson. Remember, the new postures that you will learn in this lesson are meant to be practiced every day for a week before going on to Lesson Three. Remember also that they are meant to be added to last week's basic postures, not substituted for them.

Last week, we started with the alternate stretching of the legs before getting out of bed. This you should continue to do mornings or evenings, or both. You may add to it the Toe-Twisting exercises, which help correct falling arches and even in some cases flat feet.

This exercise is very simple: Stretch out the toes of the right foot and then, without moving the foot, bend them downward, the way you would if you tried to pick up something from the floor with your toes.

Hold the toes in this position for a few seconds, then relax them. Repeat this several times. Then, instead of bending them downward, curve them upward. Hold the toes in this position for a few seconds, then relax them. Repeat this several times. Then repeat both exercises with the toes of the left foot.

Should you get a cramp while doing these or any other exercises, simply massage the affected place a little and the cramp should soon disappear. With time, you will be free of cramping altogether.

Once you are out of bed, and after having done the Rocking, which you are probably learning to enjoy for its stimulating and energizing effect, you should proceed on to the Half-Headstand. This is a simple posture that will help you prepare to do the full Headstand (Shirshasana) later on without much difficulty.

THE HALF-HEADSTAND
(Ardha Shirshasana)

Even if you have no intention of ever standing on your head, try to adopt this easy and safe upside-down position, which even babies love doing. Small children probably know instinctively what is good for them. It is good not only for them but also for you and me and anybody else who cares to try it.

We shall come to the benefits of the full Headstand in our next lesson. For the time being just try the following: Get down on your knees, clasp your hands together, interlocking your fingers, and place them together with the forearms on the floor, forming a triangle, and trying not to keep your elbows too far apart.

Place your head (about an inch above the forehead) on the mat or towel, not on your hands—cupping the palms to accommodate the head and leaving the thumbs to hold the back of your head. Now,

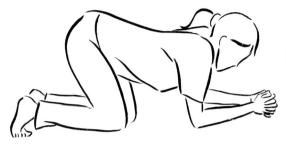

keeping your head on the floor, get up from the kneeling position, stretch your legs and stand on your toes. Then take a few small steps forward, bringing your toes as close to your head as you can.

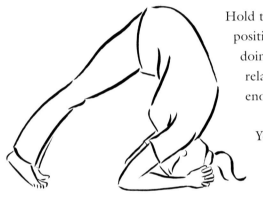

Hold this partly upside-down position for several seconds while doing deep breathing. Then relax and lie down. This is enough for your first attempt.

You have just completed the easy version of the Headstand. Did you enjoy it? It really is not too difficult, probably easier than you imagined. Often the mere thought of attempting to stand on one's head seems terrifying to beginners. "Me! Stand on my head? Never!" is what I've heard repeated again and again over the years and in all the places I have taught this discipline.

However, often only a few minutes lapsed between this "Never!" and the full Headstand actually being done. Here I must repeat, however, that you should not try this exercise more than once in a single lesson. You have a whole week's time to practice it before we try the next movement.

Caution: Do not do the Half-Headstand if your blood pressure is too high (above 150) or too low (below 100); if you get palpitations when you attempt it; if you are troubled by constipation or are going through a period of excessive dryness of the intestine; if you suffer from pus in your ears or from chronic nasal catarrh. The Headstand should also be avoided if you have organically defective pituitary, pineal, or thyroid glands, or if you feel pain in the cervical area.

THE SYMBOL OF YOGA
(Yoga Mudra)

Having taken a rest after the Half-Headstand, sit up in order to do the exercise called the Yoga Mudra, the Symbol of Yoga.

The practice of this posture is considered very important for its spiritual value in the higher stages of Yoga training when the posture is maintained for as long as one hour or more. The physical effect of the Yoga Mudra is mainly internal purification, as it helps keep our system clean by encouraging good evacuation.

In order to do the Yoga Mudra you must first sit in the Lotus Posture. If you are lucky enough to be able to assume this without practice, so much the better, but for most Occidentals this posture presents quite a problem in the beginning. However, don't let this bother you, as I will give you an easy variation of this Mudra, which you can practice until you are able to do the Lotus Posture without difficulty.

TECHNIQUE: Sit up straight on your heels. Clench your fists and place them on both sides of the abdomen, a little below the navel. Now take a deep breath and, while exhaling, bend forward as low as you can, firmly pressing your fists against the abdomen.

TIME: Remain in this position from five to ten seconds, holding your breath; then slowly straighten your back and return to the original pos-

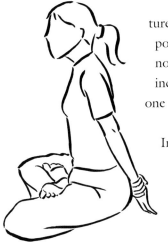

ture while you inhale. If you wish to hold this posture for a longer period of time, resume normal breathing. Eventually you should increase the time to three minutes, adding one second per week.

In order to do the Yoga Mudra in the classical manner, you should first assume the Lotus Posture. Keep both hands behind the back, clasping the left wrist with the right hand, take a deep breath and, while exhaling, bend forward until your forehead touches the floor. Remain in this posture for a few seconds, holding your breath and then slowly return to the upright position while inhaling. Take a short rest and repeat. As you keep advancing in your practice, you will find that you can hold the Yoga Mudra longer and longer. When you do, do not hold your breath any longer, but breathe deeply while maintaining this posture.

BENEFITS: The Yoga Mudra is an excellent exercise for people troubled by constipation as it increases the peristaltic movements of the bowels. It also strengthens the abdominal muscles, tones up the nervous system and the colon, and massages the pelvic region. It helps men overcome seminal weaknesses. In the higher stages of training it helps the awakening of the Kundalini, which is explained at the end of Lesson Four.

CAUTION: If you suffer from constipation, you should practice the Yoga Mudra very gently. Proceed very slowly, without any jerky movements.

Lie down on the floor and rest before going on to the next posture.

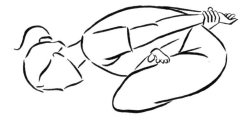

BODY-RAISING POSE
(Ardha Navasana)

This posture is also called The Boat.

TECHNIQUE: Start by lying flat on the floor. Interlock your fingers and place your hands behind your head, just above the neck. Take a deep breath, and simultaneously raise your head, shoulders and legs off the floor, without bending them. Maintain this posture for a few seconds while holding your breath, then exhale slowly while returning to the original position.

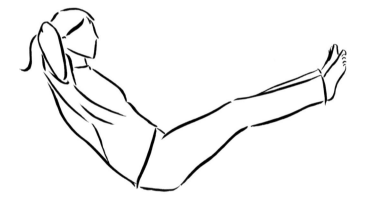

TIME: Repeat this posture. Increase the number of times gradually, from two to eight.

BENEFITS: This posture is excellent to strengthen the abdominal muscles, the pelvic region, the back and the shoulders. It helps reduce abdominal fat and relieves constipation.

CAUTION: This posture should not be done by women suffering from serious female disorders—painful menstruation or irregular periods. It should not be practiced by people with high blood pressure or severe coronary problems either.

BENDING-FORWARD POSTURE

(Hastapadasana)

After finishing the Body-Raising exercise, lie down and rest until your breathing is back to normal. Then take a few deep breaths before standing up to do the next exercise, the Bending-Forward Posture, whose Sanskrit name is Hastapadasana from hasta, which means hand, and pada, foot. As in all other postures, you will notice its English name is not a literal translation.

TECHNIQUE: Stand up straight, keeping feet together and arms hanging loosely along your sides. Inhale deeply and slide both hands from the thighs down to the ankles; then exhale. Take hold of the big toe by hooking it with the second and third fingers from inside and the thumb outside. If you cannot reach the toes, get hold of the ankles or thighs. Once you finish exhaling, try to bring your forehead to your knees without bending your legs. Hold this pose for a few seconds and then, inhaling, return to standing position, straightening the spine gently, vertebra by vertebra. Take one deep breath. Repeat this exercise twice.

Here is another version of the same posture. Place your hands on the floor, palms up, and then step on your fingertips with your toes. Straighten, or try straightening your legs, pressing your head against them.

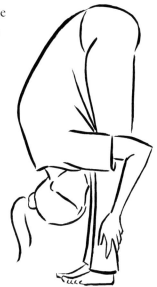

TIME: Remain in this posture from two to ten seconds. At the beginning do only twice, gradually increasing up to five. Ultimately you will be able to hold this posture while breathing in a normal way.

BENEFITS: The Bending-Forward Posture is a very invigorating exercise. It gives buoyancy to the body, removes abdominal fat and flabbiness, and relieves constipation and gas. It also gives a good pull to the sciatic nerves and makes knees straight.

CAUTION: This posture should be done very slowly, without any jerkiness. After finishing it you can lie down for a moment, if you wish, or proceed with the next posture.

It must not be practiced by people with cardiac problems and high blood pressure, nor is it advisable in cases of hiatal hernia, as well as when there are stomachaches. People suffering from dizziness should also refrain from practicing it.

FOOTLIFT POSE (THE STORK)
(Ardha Baddha Pada Uttanasana): First Movement

Next you will try the first version of the Footlift Pose. Its Sanskrit name is such a long one, Ardha Baddha Pada Uttanasana, that we nick-named it "The Stork."

TECHNIQUE: Stand up straight and raise the left foot, bending the knees. Using both hands, place the left foot on the right thigh, as high as you can. Hold it there with the right hand. Keep the knee down to the level of the right knee so that it does not stick out. Your spine should be erect. Stand steady on the right foot as long as possible and do one deep breathing. Repeat the exercise with your right foot up on the left thigh.

Of course, to remain standing steady for as long as possible is easier said than done. Usually during the first days one does everything but stand still—hopping around on one leg and desperately trying to grasp something for support. But don't feel discouraged: it can be done.

As I have said before, this is the first version of the Footlift Pose. At this stage it serves only to develop balance. In the next lesson you will learn the second movement of this posture. In the meantime, lie down and relax before going on to the next posture.

REVERSE POSTURE
(Viparita Karani Mudra)

The next exercise will be the Reverse Posture. In Sanskrit it is called Viparita Karani Mudra. The Asanas, or postures, are supposed to give strength, while the Mudras, or gestures, are supposed to give balance and steadiness.

According to the yogis, "the sun dwells at the root of the navel (the solar plexus), and the moon at the root of the palate." In the Reverse Posture the position is reversed and the sun rises above the moon.

TECHNIQUE: This posture is hardly difficult to assume by most people. Simply lie down on your back, take a deep breath and raise both legs and buttocks off the floor. While doing this, quickly put your hands on your hips to support yourself. Keep your thumbs just under the hipbone and place your elbows on the floor, about a foot apart. If the elbows are too wide apart they will not give adequate support to the body, which should be resting on them. Do not bend the knees; keep your legs straight and stretch your feet, but don't strain yourself. Close your eyes and remain in this position while doing deep breathing, even if you feel a little uncomfortable in the beginning.

TIME: At first keep this posture for ten seconds, gradually increasing its duration by five seconds until you reach two minutes.

BENEFITS: The Reverse Posture is considered a restorer of youth and vitality. It keeps the glands, organs, and skin in a youthful condition, erases premature wrinkles and delays aging. This posture is especially recommended for women who suffer from sexual disorders, or have irregular or painful periods; it also relieves the physical and mental discomforts during menopause.

It is said that the practice of this mudra preserves or restores manly vigor. It affects partly the thyroid gland, but mainly the gonads or sexual glands, which control the aging processes in our bodies.

The Reverse Posture is very popular in various beauty centers and gyms, but it is seldom accompanied by deep breathing.

If for any reason you are afraid of practicing this posture or believe it is beyond your capabilities, try it at first with the aid of a table, and you will be surprised to find that you can do it easily in just a few minutes. Do as follows:

Sit down on the floor with your legs extended under the table and your forehead touching the edge of the table; now lie down on your back, raise both legs to the height of the table and press the middle of your soles against the table's edge, so that your heels are below the edge and your toes above it. Now lift your buttocks and support your body with both hands, holding your back at waist level and keeping your elbows firmly placed on the floor. Remain in this position for a short while and breathe deeply. Then slowly try to straighten first one leg and then the other. It will be easier if you first carry your legs a little towards your head, rather than keep them perfectly straight while you are not able yet to do so.

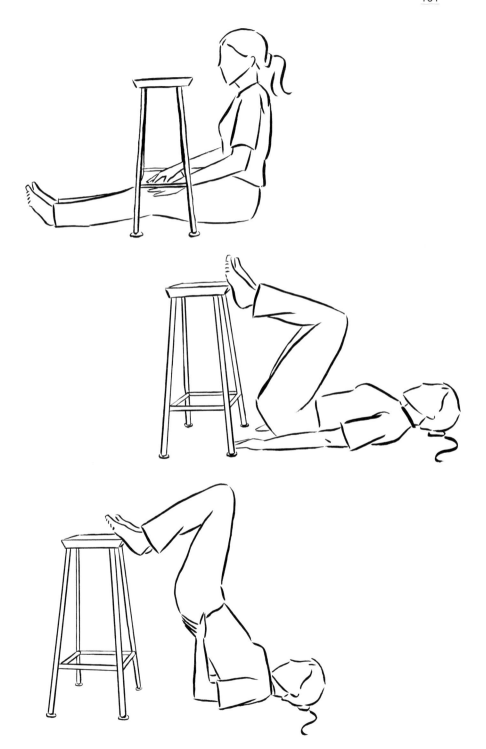

After finishing this posture lie down and take a short rest. Then get up to practice the breathing exercises.

Breathing Exercises

BREATHING EXERCISE FOR GOOD POSTURE

Stand straight with feet together. Put your hands behind your back and interlock the fingers, palms upwards. This movement will make your elbows twist automatically.

Inhale deeply, then bend forward while exhaling, at the same time raising the arms until they are completely stretched upwards. Do not bend them, but keep them straight throughout. Lower your head and try to raise your arms even more. Remain for a moment in this position, holding your breath; then slowly return to the original point while exhaling and keeping fingers interlocked. Repeat this exercise two or three times.

Another version is done kneeling in the Diamond Position or Vajrasana, as shown in the following pictures. The steps are the same, except here you bend over until your forehead touches the floor.

This is an excellent exercise for the waistline or for relieving weak backs, but especially for stooped shoulders. It should be taught to all children at home and at school to counteract their tendency to slouch, for slouching, in addition to being ugly, develops a bad and unhealthy posture as it prevents the lungs from expanding as they should.

If people could only see for themselves how ugly and apathetic bad posture makes them look, they would quickly get to work to correct it. This is especially true of women who wear very tight dresses with bare backs.

I am reminded of an incident on the street in Honolulu: a lovely young woman took off her stole in front of me, suddenly baring a shockingly unattractive back with bones protruding out like wings. A little later, the same thing happened to me at the beach. The friends I was with got ready to go into the water and I suddenly saw they all had these kinds of "wings." I looked around me and realized that was the norm, and was able to observe that there were very few women or even young girls with a straight spine, and therefore a beautiful, dignified bearing. As soon as I got to my room, I took a small mirror and started to observe my own back. I can say I didn't see any problem with it. However, I am absolutely sure that years ago, before I started to practice Yoga exercises, I would have felt dismayed looking at it, since I myself used to have that awful habit of slouching, much to my mother's mortification; she was always after me to stand up and walk straight.

Rhythmic Breathing

And now, before we finish this lesson with a little rest and relaxation, you will learn rhythmic breathing.

In India, they say that by practicing rhythmic breathing you become attuned to the rhythm of the Universe; and that by establishing direct contact with the whole world you come to experience a sense of oneness with it. Then the feeling of separateness and isolation disappears and with it fear, loneliness, frustration, doubt, despair, and other dismal states of mind.

If practiced properly, rhythmic breathing, as well as concentration and meditation—which we shall see in our last lesson—may bring about a huge change in both the physical as well as the mental state of someone, and serve as a step toward spiritual evolution. Through rhythmic breathing one also becomes aware of one's own breathing. Each individual functions according to a personal rhythm, his or her own tempo, and when thrown off, whether by a nervous breakdown, any intense emotion, a taxing job, or strained family or business relationships, a person loses his or her inner equilibrium. If the situation continues this way and a person does not recover the inner balance, he or she becomes a nervous wreck or ends up in a state of collapse. The practice of rhythmic breathing can undoubtedly avert or remedy many of these unhappy situations.

Rhythmic breathing can help a person acquire self-confidence, optimism, mental serenity, and many other desired qualities. The power one develops with it is neither positive nor negative—it simply is. It is up to us to use it for good or evil. We must be very careful never to make bad use of it.

TECHNIQUE: Rhythmic breathing is practiced in the same way as deep breathing, but it is timed to the rhythm of your heartbeat. Inhalation and exhalation should be done regularly, in order to establish an even rhythm.

Sit down in the Lotus Pose or, if uncomfortable, get into a crossed-legged position or sit on a chair. The important thing is to keep your spine very straight. Do not forget to undo your belt or bra, or loosen up your tie, if you are wearing any of these items. Keep your back straight, and put your hands on your knees as you start to take a few deep breaths. Now put your index finger, middle and ring fingers of your right hand on your left wrist to find the pulse. Listen carefully to the beats and start counting 1, 2, 3, 4 several times, following the heartbeats.

Continue mentally counting 1, 2, 3, 4—1, 2, 3, 4 until you fall into this rhythm and can follow it without holding your pulse. Then put your hands on your knees and take a deep breath while counting 1, 2; then exhale while counting once more 1, 2, 3, 4.

Repeat two or three times, no more. This is rhythmic breathing.

Should four beats be too much for you, count only to three. If they are too few, you may count to five or six while inhaling, and the same while exhaling. When breathing in, do not stop at the end of the count, that is, try not to have extra time to finish inhaling: adjust your breathing so that both inhalation and exhalation become rhythmic and have no gaps in between. Inhalation and exhalation should always take an equal time to do.

TIME: You may repeat this exercise again in the evening but do not overdo it at the beginning. Start by practicing it three or four times, adding one each week until you finally reach the desired number, which may be sixty or more.

Posture for Meditation

There are several classical postures for meditation.

If the Lotus position is too difficult for you, you may try the Accomplished Pose, called the Siddhasana in Sanskrit. Siddha means adept or accomplished yogi. It is done as follows:

Sit down with both legs outstretched. Bend the left one and place the left foot sole against the right thigh, so that the heel touches the perineum. Then bend the right knee and place the right heel against the pubic bone. With thumb and index fingers together, form a circle in what is called the Gnani Mudra. Keep your hands on your knees with palms upwards if you practice this exercise between sunrise and sunset; after sunset reverse the palms. The spine should always be perfectly erect.

Here is another classic posture for meditation. It is called Swastikasana in Sanskrit. Sit on the exercise mat, bend the right leg and put the sole of the right foot against the left thigh, so that the heel is against the groin. Now bend the left knee and place the left foot toes between the right thigh and calf. Hold the spine straight. Place your hands as in the Accomplished Pose.

Still another is the Symmetrical Pose, or Samasana in Sanskrit. The only difference between this posture and the previous one is the position of the heels: in the Swastikasana both heels press against the opposite groins, whereas here both heels should be set against the pubic bone—first the right, then the left. The toes of the right foot are pushed under the left thigh and those of the left foot are placed on the right calf, with the sole upturned. The spine and hands are kept in the same position as in the previous postures. If you cannot assume any of these postures for the time being, choose a comfortable position in which your head and back are in one straight line.

The Diet

It is from the mastery based on the liberty to choose between the satisfaction of the appetites and the flight toward Spirituality that human dignity is born.

—LECOMTE DU NOÜY, Human Destiny[1]

The colon is the mirror of mind—when the mind gets right, the colon gets right.

—SWAMI PARAMANANDA,
Concentration and Meditation[2]

No course in Yoga can be considered complete without making reference to the diet, so let us go over some of its most essential aspects.

We all know that, after air and water, food is essential to keep our bodies healthy, young and strong. Doesn't it seem like a paradox that it is in the U.S., the richest country in the world, that people suffer most from malnutrition and bad eating habits, in the midst of so much abundance?

According to the leading scientists and nutritionists, one of the main causes for this is overeating; the other is eating the wrong kinds of food. Our organism is nourished only by those foods it is capable of breaking down and assimilating. Food that is not properly digested turns into poison for our body. Foods that are excessively devitalized, artificial and unwholesome are what the American population most consumes. The result is that our health picture looks more and more dismal. Diseases, especially degenerative diseases, are reaching such proportions that even people who are apparently healthy, or believed to be so, if tested carefully reveal some hidden ailment, which one day unexpectedly sends them to a hospital bed, an operating table, or a grave.

Often, we hear that one or another of our friends has suddenly developed diabetes, asthma, arthritis, or some other degenerative disease. We also frequently read in the newspapers about people who are taken suddenly to a mental hospital or drop dead of a sudden heart attack in the prime of life—usually between the ages of forty-five and fifty-five, although apparently there had been nothing wrong with them previously. But the truth is, this kind of ailment is rarely sudden; in all probability it is the fatal result of many years of poison accumulation due to an inadequate lifestyle or wrong eating habits.

Reading such news may frighten us, yet what do we do to prevent them from happening again? At best, we decide upon a physical checkup, but even if we do get around to doing it, which seldom happens, few times do we actually resolve to change our living and eating habits. In spite of the many warnings constantly appearing in various newspapers, books and magazines, not to mention health publications, we simply follow the same routine as usual.

By way of example here are just a few relevant quotes that confirm my way of thinking and that of so many others:

POOR DIET LINKED TO MENTAL ILLNESS

According to a group of nutrition specialists, inadequate eating is the cause of a great many illnesses.

An adequate diet is not only an effective remedy for any ailment related to blood pressure, but also for many mental illnesses. . . . The slowing down of the metabolic processes (changing food into energy, tissue and body secretion) is caused by poor diet—too much white sugar and flour and not enough fruits, vegetables, meat and milk.

EATING RELATED TO GALLSTONES

One out of three cases of gall bladder trouble may be cured without surgery, according to the Minnesota State Medical Association.

This association insists that a quiet life and a daily control of food intake, as well as a change in the patients' habits and exercise, can accomplish a great deal for the one adult in five who has gallstones.

BURNING UP FAT

The elements utilized to produce most gallstones are made when the body burns fat. The way the body burns fat depends in turn on the glands, just as the amount of fat to be burned depends on the diet. If anything is wrong with either, gallstones are likely to form.

To stay clear of gallstones, the association suggests drinking eight or more glasses of water each day, eat plenty of fat-free meat and avoid ice-cold drinks. Also avoid too much fried food, salad dressing, butter, oil and cream. They suggest eating fruit three times a day.

DOCTOR SEES DIET AND CANCER TIE-UP

Dr. E. Vincent Coudry, of Hope Medical Center, said that by reducing the intake of calories the incidence of cancer is also reduced. During World War II in Germany and other occupied countries the reduction of cancer cases was very marked because people were on low-calorie diets.[3]

It is interesting to note that in his work *The Cancer Therapy*, Dr. Max Gerson also speaks of fifty cancer cases cured, thanks to a special diet based on fresh vegetables, fruits and juices, without any salt or proteins. He emphasizes that the juice must be freshly squeezed and immediately consumed, that is, no more than ten or fifteen minutes after it has been squeezed; otherwise, it loses its enzymes—the minute particles that are carriers of vital energy in our bodies.

This is a good opportunity to remind you that the juice of vegetables and fruits grown in organically treated soil is tremendously richer in enzymes than that from produce raised in chemically treated soil. I have seen this fact conclusively demonstrated by means of the Nemeoscope, so far the only existing instrument that is able to project on a screen the resolution of the enzymes and show them in their uniform structure and in action.

"Our Starving Teenagers" is the title of a dramatic article that once appeared in *Reader's Digest,* and was subsequently reprinted for distribution in separate leaflet form. This article dealt with malnutrition among teenagers who have not yet reached twenty, a phenomenon that has become nationwide. They fill up on empty calories from food that is supposed to satiate their hunger—hamburgers, french fries, candy bars and soft drinks—leaving no room for healthy, nutritious food. The result: the deteriorating health and weakening of our future world population.

And there is something even more serious: most of the damage is permanent. It affects not only the offenders but also their future children: "What a woman eats during the period of pregnancy and nursing directly affects the intelligence of her child."[4]

Another news item reads as follows:

ANIMAL FAT DIET BLAMED FOR HEART ILLS INCREASE

"A diet high in animal fats is the villain in the mounting rate of heart and blood vessel diseases," according to Dr. C. M. Wilhelmj of the Creighton School of Medicine. ". . . A normal diet of a well-to-do family today is from fifty to sixty-eight percent fat. Our diets have been going higher in fat content the last twenty to thirty years, so has our rate of heart and blood vessel diseases."[5]

When you consider the daily food intake of a normal healthy adult should not contain more than twenty to thirty percent fat, including fat derived from eggs, dairy products, nuts and baked foods, it is small wonder that doctors worry so much about the nation's eating habits. Another important factor to consider is not only the quantity of fat, but its quality. Unsaturated fats, mostly derived from plants and oils, are regarded as essential because they are low in cholesterol. The best sources of these are sunflower seed oil, soybean oil, corn oil and sesame seed oil. Saturated fats, mostly derived from animals, eggs and dairy products, are regarded as unessential as they are high in cholesterol. Animal products with the highest concentration of cholesterol are the brain, liver and egg yolk; those with the lowest cholesterol are milk, cottage cheese and fish. All fruits and most vegetables are low in cholesterol.

Unsaturated fatty acids move about swiftly in our organism, whereas the saturated settle and become deposits. Professor G. J. Shoepfer, of the University of Minnesota Hospitals, Minneapolis, reports[6] that even one meal with too much saturated fat can cause a heart attack in a susceptible person. Also:

> At the 20th session of the American Academy of Nutrition Dr. Eugene H. Payne said that cooking fats like lard and butter, which are popular in the United States, England, Sweden, and Holland, cause in these countries more deaths from circulatory diseases than any other illness. "Excess fat leads to premature degeneration of the liver, heart, kidneys, and blood vessels. . . . Putting on weight, that is, an increase in fat tissue, should be considered a serious metabolic disorder, even if the individual still feels healthy. . . . Fat is continuously in circulation; that is: some is put away in storage but, at the same time, storage fat is again put into circulation. Continuous turnover is a sign of health; with reduced turnover, metabolic disorder begins."[7]

I could go on quoting report after report from newspapers, medical journals, magazines and books. There are more and more articles every day of this kind. However, in spite of so many serious warnings, most people still think there is nothing wrong with their diet. "We always eat this way" is what they usually argue.

Probably because the damaging effects of an improper diet do not produce immediate ill results, we seldom blame our diet for our increasing ailments. How many people are there who, in spite of being well informed on this cultural change, would attribute a cold, fever, asthma, arthritis, heart problems and mental disorders to a toxic condition? Very few. Fewer still are those who correct their eating habits, go on a cleansing diet or a fast, or practice deep breathing in order to get more oxygen when they need it to remain healthy.

For some strange reason, even constipation is rarely linked with a faulty diet, although so many of our physical troubles originate in the stomach. Many of us might well join in a little prayer inscribed at the entrance to a fifteenth-century cathedral in Chester, England, which reads, "O Lord, give me a good digestion, but also something to digest." Maybe we should also pray for fewer things to digest.

Dr. Ehrenfried E. Pfeiffer, Professor of Nutrition at Farleigh-Dickinson University, said in one of his lectures that to develop and keep up good health, "one has to maintain a balanced diet which must be planned before the food enters the mouth." In other words, you must first decide upon the menu and then proceed to consume it.

It is not easy to suggest a diet that suits everyone, since a diet is a very personal matter. Much depends upon each person's physical condition, morphological structure, weight, height, age and even occupation and lifestyle. The food intake of a brain worker who is confined to a desk would, for instance, be inadequate for someone who does hard labor or works with his hands; the same can be said about a pregnant woman who is about to give birth: she can hardly thrive on the menu of a dieting model. Moreover, as one ages, not only the amount but also the type of food varies. The quantity and quality of food needed for a baby, a child, a teenager, an adult, and an older person are completely different.

In Dr. Ehrenfried E. Pfeiffer's *Balanced Nutrition, Know What You Eat and Why*, we read that during the period of growth one needs more calories in one's diet, with a large amount of carbohydrates, which should be well balanced. The adult between twenty-five and forty-two needs fewer calories, fewer carbohydrates and more proteins, which should also be well calculated. With maturity, not as many calories are needed, the diet should be lower in fat, and proteins should be prevalent.

But even within the same age bracket there are fluctuations. There are people who are old at forty, while others are just starting to live at this age. My own mother at seventy-seven looked like a fifty-five-year-old woman and felt that age. She practiced her Yoga exercises every day, including the Headstand; ran the household, danced at parties and kept the clear and strong voice of a young woman.

In order to determine what to eat and what not to eat, you must study your own particular situation and then begin experimenting with various foods and combinations of foods to find out what suits you best. Remember: one man's food is another man's poison! Only, please don't turn into a food nut who talks of nothing but his meals, digestion and elimination. Avoid trying foods by mistake or without thinking, like that man I once saw at a health lecture, who kept loudly agreeing with everything the nutritionist was saying while gorging on cheap candy bars. When, unable to suppress a smile, I suggested that he was doing the exact opposite of what the speaker was preaching, the man grinned sheepishly, showing a row of shockingly bad teeth, and said apologetically: "I am only experimenting!"

Health lectures in the United States have done much to make the public diet-conscious, but they are also responsible for causing considerable confusion with their contradictory theories. One theory recommends drinking large amounts of milk; the next thunders against it. One is all for raw foods; the next thunders against them. There are those who advise eating meat, while others totally condemn it. And so it goes on, until the poor listener is so mixed up he returns to his old—and generally bad—eating habits.

There are, however, a few "musts" on which almost everybody does agree. Personally, I learned them from my Yoga teacher in India, Sri Krishnamacharya, who lived to be 101 years old. They are: Do not overeat; avoid dead foods; eat a lot of fresh fruits, salads, and vegetables, or fruit and vegetable juices, provided you don't suffer from any ailment where raw food is prohibited; drink lots of fresh water during the day, and, finally, breathe a sufficient quantity of fresh air.

The best foods—those that are pure, fresh, clean and natural, such as vegetables, greens, fruits, whole grains, honey, the oils already mentioned, nuts, milk, eggs, fish and meat—contain all necessary vitamins, minerals, amino acids, enzymes, and the vital chemical substances that control our metabolism. Remember that metabolism is the pulse of life.

The "dead" foods are those that have been robbed of their natural vitamins, minerals, amino acids and enzymes by processing of different kinds. They include products that have been canned, preserved, pickled, bottled, bleached, polished, refined and otherwise devitalized. White flour, white rice and white sugar belong in this category, since they have been bleached, polished and refined almost to nothing as far as nutritious value. They should be replaced in the diet by whole grain flour, brown rice, and raw sugar—but not white sugar mixed with molasses to color it and then sold as "brown sugar."

The best sweetener is natural honey, obtained from private bee-owners or bought at health-food stores. The label will tell you whether it has been heated or processed, that is, "if anything has been added or taken away." Here is what one German scientist has discovered about this kind of honey:

HONEY EATING GETS SUPPORT

"The West German Research Society has discovered that thousands of years ago Roman wrestlers ate large quantities of honey to increase their fighting strength. Now they have heard that Russian athletes regularly eat honey for the same reason. As a result, the society is advocating eating more honey, only it emphasizes that it should be in its natural state, rather than heated up to make it keep longer."

So much for honey. As for white sugar, the dental authority Dr. Melvin E. Page explains in his book, *Body Chemistry in Health and Disease,* how white sugar disturbs the sugar-calcium-phosphorus balance in the body. As a result it leads to dental decay. And while on the subject of tooth decay, let us mention that starches, too, help create favorable conditions for it by affecting the saliva in the mouth.

Another adverse effect of white sugar is that it interferes with the maintenance of a balanced blood-sugar level, thus robbing the system of vitamin B. Long before the development of the Salk vaccine in 1948, another medical authority, Dr. Benjamin F. Sandler, author of *Diet Prevents Polio,* was able to check a polio epidemic threatening North Carolina by advising parents over the radio not to give children candy in any form until the danger was over. Thus he had discovered the link between the intake of soft drinks and sugar, and polio.

White flour, which is a concentrated carbohydrate, is converted to sugar in the liver. The bleaching and processing deprive it of its natural vitamins and minerals. Therefore all foods made of this flour, such as bread, noodles, cakes, cookies, pies, soups and gravies, have very little nutritional value and are mainly "empty calories."

In her book *Feel Like a Million*, Catharyn Elwood tells of a group of school children who were preparing an exhibit of mice for a fair in Long Beach. Some mice were fed on puffed wheat and some on whole grain wheat. A few days before the fair opened, the puffed-wheat-fed mice died, and the youngsters then and there refused to eat puffed wheat at home.

Let me also mention an experiment made in school with a human tooth: The tooth was dropped into a bottle containing one of the most popular soft drinks. Within three weeks it had completely dissolved. Only then did the youngsters understand why the school authorities had prohibited the sale of soft drinks on the grounds.

According to a sportsman from Finland some years ago, the Russian Olympic team members owed their physical fitness to their nutritious food and special breathing exercises. In an interview given to the Swiss magazine *Volksgesundheit* around that time, this same Finn said that while he was trying to find out the real reason for the huge success of the Russians in the Olympics, he began observing them closely during the games in Helsinki and Falun. A perfect knowledge of their language allowed him to engage in friendly conversation with his Russian colleagues and to spend a great deal of time with them. According to the Finn, they had two great advantages over the other participants in the sports. First, they used a special breathing technique that enabled them to feel at ease and rested while all the rest were puffing and panting. The second was their healthy lifestyle and natural diet based on organic foods that mainly consisted of fresh vegetables, greens, fruits, and milk products. All these were of a quality unfortunately unobtainable in the "civilized" Occidental countries, as fruits and vegetables in Russia were still raised at that time in healthy soil treated with natural fertilizers, not with chemical ones. Consequently, milk, too, came from healthy cows whose grass and fodder were not grown with the help of chemicals.

By the way, we should point out that vegetables fertilized with chemicals are overly rich in potassium and exceedingly poor in magnesium;

this imbalance produces toxicity in the human body. But the majority of the Russians were not familiar yet with the craze for technically poisoning natural foods. The Finnish sportsman to whom we were referring concluded by saying that his findings should help orient not only all sportsmen in the world, but also all other people the world over to do some serious thinking on this subject.

Judging from the *Volksgesundheit* article, the diet of the Russian athletes is very similar to that recommended by Indian yogis. Both give ample proof of the truly amazing results of a natural organic diet combined with special breathing techniques and a healthy lifestyle backed up by exercising. A remarkable example of this is the Hunzas of India. These people have caught the attention of the world because of their exceptional good health and longevity. Men of more than a hundred years old are still strong enough to do heavy work and till the soil, and their teeth show no signs of decay. I myself have seen almost miraculous transformations and recoveries in people who have taken up the practice of Yoga and changed their eating habits. This includes my own case.

On our pantry shelves at home you will never find anything canned, preserved, bottled, bleached, refined or processed. Whole grain flour substitutes for white flour; brown rice takes the place of white rice; honey replaces white sugar for table and kitchen use. Cocoa and chocolate are also absent in our pantry, and carob powder is used in our desserts and beverages. Personally I don't care for desserts and generally drink coffee substitutes made from toasted grain, fruits or toasted cereals, or various herb teas, skim milk, fresh fruit and vegetable juices and a large amount of fresh water with or without lemon. We also use lemons instead of vinegar. For seasoning foods we utilize all kinds of vegetable, mineral and sea salts, soy sauce, as well as fresh and dry herbs, onion and garlic. Onion and garlic, by the way, were forbidden by my Yoga teacher for the duration of my training, just as were all other vegetables that do not ripen under the direct rays of the sun, such as beets, carrots, radishes and potatoes. The reason for this is that during the period of apprenticeship, the disciple should remain chaste and, for such, he must avoid all passion-inducing foods.

It goes without saying that, as a Yoga disciple, I was not able to touch alcohol, cigarettes or meat, none of which made any difference to me, since I was already abstemious, a vegetarian and a non-smoker. But I liked coffee, which I also gave up, along with tea, chocolate and cocoa, because my teacher considered them poisonous.

Alcohol is avoided by the yogis because it lowers the vibrations of the astral body, whereas the purpose of Yoga is to heighten these vibrations. They do not smoke, because tobacco congests and poisons lungs, and Yoga's purpose is to clean all organs in the human body. Smoking is also supposed to damage and reduce the astral web to breaking point, which in a developed individual should be thin and strong enough to protect him from the lower influences. Meat is not eaten for several reasons. To begin with, yogis don't believe in killing for any reason at all, but on top of that, the idea of eating something dead is absolutely repulsive to them. The astral vibrations of the slaughtered animal have an effect on the astral body of the person eating that meat.

One of our friends, a university professor from Europe, had to give up eating meat because he started seeing the astral bodies of the killed animals he was about to eat. He told me, for instance, that oysters, scallops and crabs, so rich in protein, were the worst for our own astral bodies and fish the least harmful.

However, you don't need to exclude from your diet all these foods, since you are not subject to the strict disciplines of a Yoga disciple and can make your own choices. If you do smoke, you should at least do the deep breathing exercises to keep your lungs cleaner and healthier.

In order to obtain better results from these teachings you should go over, for your own benefit, your eating habits. Every person in the

Western world would profit from adopting a more sensible and balanced diet than the present one, for our eating habits are slowly but surely damaging the health of the population. So if you are anxious to regain or reestablish your lost youth and retain it, don't neglect the following diet suggestions to which I personally adhere in my daily life.

1) Never drink iced water, especially during meals, as this interferes with the free course of digestive juices and makes digestion difficult. Drinking iced water is a sin against proper digestion and you must not give in to this bad habit.

2) Drink a glass of fresh, pure water at room temperature, as soon as you wake up in the morning and when going to bed at night. It should be taken hot when one is constipated. In this case, a little lemon may be added. Hot water, or herb tea with lemon—and honey if you wish—taken on a hot summer day will make you feel cooler afterward.

3) Drink from five to eight glasses of water every day, or one glass for every fourteen pounds of your body weight. In countries where fluoride is added to the water, drink distilled water to be on the safe side. Next to air, water is one of the main elements most urgently demanded by human beings. Eight-tenths of our physical body is made of water and we eliminate about two quarts of it a day. An insufficient intake of water is often the cause of constipation and a congested colon, as well as a defective functioning of the liver and kidneys, and of clogged bowels.

4) Don't drink water with your meals, but take it half an hour before or two to three hours after meals so it does not disturb the digestion process by diluting digestive juices.

5) Sip water slowly; never gulp it all at once.

6) In order to restore to water the vital elements lost during boiling or processing, pass it through the air, pouring it from one glass into

another several times. You will soon note that this produces a slightly invigorating and stimulating effect on the organism, which is absent in lifeless and devitalized water.

7) It is better to eat fruit rather than to drink fruit juices. When you prepare fresh juices with such vegetables as carrots, radishes, beets, etc., add some of the juice from other vegetables that grow out in the air and the sun.

8) Don't keep juices for later, as they will lose their rich enzymes.

9) Orange juice, for instance, loses one-third of them after half an hour of being squeezed, and all juices lose their enzymes after two hours.

10) Alcohol, tea, coffee, cocoa and chocolate are not recommended, because tannic acid, theine, caffeine and theobromine are stimulants.

11) Milk is a food, not a drink. It should be taken in small sips, other-wise it is likely to produce indigestion.

12) It is not the amount of food you eat that nourishes your body, but the quantity the body itself can assimilate.

13) Choose carefully the foods that suit your system; choose them with the same care as you select your clothes. At the beginning, you will have to experiment, trying different foods and various combina-tions until you find out which suit you best.

14) Avoid all kinds of devitalized foods, such as canned goods, white rice, white flour and white sugar. Eat whole wheat, whole-wheat flour and brown sugar or honey. Try to cut down on candy, pastries, and vinegar, except cider vinegar.

15) Chew your food carefully, especially if it belongs to the starchy

group, so that it mixes well with saliva. Unless converted into glucose by the saliva in the mouth, starch will lie rotting in the stomach for several hours.

16) Toasted or dry bread is better than fresh, but do not eat bread together with any liquid, because it is important to let the teeth work on it properly. Better have whatever you want to drink before eating the bread, as starch should be converted into glucose by the saliva.

17) Eat only one starch to a meal. For instance, if you take rice omit bread, potatoes, spaghetti, pudding, gravy, etc.

18) If you suffer from gas, it is advisable to plan your meals so that you do not eat starch and protein together, and especially not with cooked sulfur foods like peas, cabbage, cauliflower, eggs, turnips and so on, because gas is produced by sulfur working on starch. See the Hay Diet in Appendix I.

19) Don't throw away the water in which vegetables have been boiled, but use it for soup, gravies, or for drinking. Potato water is very good as it alkalizes the body. See recipe in Appendix I.

20) Don't throw away the peels of carrots or beets (these should be cooked first or scalded with boiling water before cooking); add them to the soup tied in a bundle, then throw them away after the soup is cooked.

21) Vegetables should be cooked in very little water, over slow fire, or better still without any water, in special vapor-sealing stainless steel pans.

22) Fried foods should be avoided altogether, because they digest even slower than fat itself. Fat is the last element to leave the stomach; carbohydrates are the ones to go first and next are proteins.

23) All saturated fats, such as butter, margarine, eggs and dairy products,

tend to increase the blood cholesterol level and can be classified as nonessential fat.

24) Highest in cholesterol are brains, egg yolk and liver; the lowest are milk, cottage cheese, and fish. All fruit and most vegetables are also low in cholesterol.

25) Any diet with a high content of saturated fat is dangerous. You should eat balanced foods: a high-fat and low-protein diet inhibits the enzymes' functioning.

26) All unsaturated fats such as oils keep the blood cholesterol level low and can be classified as essential fats. The best sources are sunflower seed oil, soybean oil, sesame seed oil, and cornflower oil.

27) Remember that good nutrition and health are not only about calories and the amount of fat, but about the quality of fat. Bacon, for instance, has caloric fat value only. It contains nothing else, neither vitamins, nor minerals.

28) Warming up meals containing fat of any kind, oil included, renders them more and more indigestible with each reheating. Both deep-frying and reusing fat left in the frying pan are not recommended either for the same reason. Try to use only oils labeled "cold pressed," usually obtainable in health food stores.

29) Any of the oils mentioned in paragraph 27, as well as the old-fashioned cod liver oil, are very good lubricants for the system and contribute to better elimination if taken at night; take one tablespoon three to four hours after the last meal.

30) Six glasses of fresh green cabbage juice a day keep peptic ulcers away.

31) One of the best tonics is the so-called "Calcium Cocktail." According to Professor Carl Albin, calcium, lemon, sulfur (the egg yolk), honey and a little alcohol, all mixed together, restore the normal

balance and activity of the gonads, or sexual glands, within thirty to sixty days. It is prepared as follows: Put eight raw eggs into a jar, without breaking their shells. (The eggs should be fertile and must come from chickens that are allowed to run free. The commercially distributed eggs lack certain vitamins.) Today you can get ecological eggs in some specialized stores. Cover the eggs with the juice of sixteen lemons, preferably grown organically without any poisonous spray on them, and keep in refrigerator for four to six days, until shells are dissolved by the lemon and reduced to powder. Take out the eggs, being careful not to break the thin membrane, separate the yolks from the whites—which are not used—and put the yolks back into the bowl. Press its contents through a sieve or put into a food processor, add raw honey to taste and pour in two to three ounces of brandy. Keep in refrigerator. Take a tablespoonful three times a day before meals, shaking well before using. Even though I am abstemious, I recommend preparing this recipe with the brandy, since the alcohol is supposed to extract the active ingredients. It also acts as a natural stabilizer.

32) The richest source of protein is the soybean. Two pounds of soybean flour contain as much protein as four pounds of cheese, five pounds of boneless meat, six dozen eggs, or fifteen quarts of milk. Soybean is the only non-acid-forming protein. For more on this subject, read *Soybeans for Health, Longevity and Economy* by Dr. Philip S. Chen, published by Chemical Elements.

Apart from the many instructions issued in these articles, the main rule about food is that together with the quantity, quality and preparation of it, the mental attitude at the time of eating is of great importance.

Aside from the fact that you should never eat in a hurry, it is of vital importance that the act of nourishing yourself be a joyful one, taken in good company and in pleasant circumstances. Food eaten in a state of anger, irritation or nervousness produces a toxic condition in the body. Therefore, it is better to skip a meal when this is the case and wait until you recover your peace of mind.

Try to make your mealtime a harmonious moment, avoiding unpleasant discussions. An attractively set table also adds to the pleasure of eating. So does a smiling face, a cheerful word, a beautiful flower or a picture. Bless your food and enjoy it.

You should never break unpleasant news immediately after a meal or at the table, because you not only upset digestion but the entire organism. You will understand the reason perfectly well when you get to the third lesson, in which we will talk about stress and the elements that cause it.

1. New York: Longmans, Green & Co., Inc., 1947.
2. Cohasset, Mass.: The Vedanta Centre.
3. Chris Clauson in the *Los Angeles Examiner,* November 29, 1955.
4. Columbi Teacher's Report, released in 1955.
5. Associated Press, Omaha, Nebraska, March 10, 1955.
6. *The New England Journal of Medicine,* December 26, 1957.
7. The *Los Angeles Times,* May 21, 1956.

Lesson Three • Third Week

Mind is the master of senses and
breath is the master of mind.
The mind cannot be restrained
without restraining the breath—
mental activity keeps pace with respiration.

HEADSTAND
(Shirshasana): First Stage

After practicing the Half-Headstand for a whole week, you should be ready to try the full Headstand, or Shirshasana. By far the simplest, safest approach for the beginner is to try the posture first in a corner, in order to have maximum support. When you attempt the Headstand this way, you don't need to feel either nervous or insecure, for the walls afford protection on both sides and exclude the possibility of falling.

However, you will need a helping hand to help you stand on your head the first few times. Anyone can help you; no special skill is needed. A friend of mine who lives by herself and is the kind of person who hesitates to ask for help told me she managed her very first headstand completely alone: she pushed an armchair to the corner of the

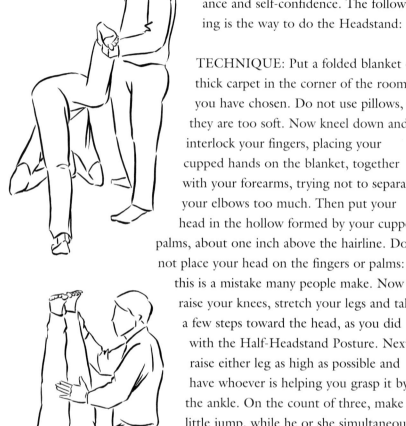

room, then put her leg on the arm of the chair while managing to practice the posture. This was the procedure she chose until she had acquired a sense of balance and self-confidence. The following is the way to do the Headstand:

TECHNIQUE: Put a folded blanket or thick carpet in the corner of the room you have chosen. Do not use pillows, as they are too soft. Now kneel down and interlock your fingers, placing your cupped hands on the blanket, together with your forearms, trying not to separate your elbows too much. Then put your head in the hollow formed by your cupped palms, about one inch above the hairline. Do not place your head on the fingers or palms: this is a mistake many people make. Now raise your knees, stretch your legs and take a few steps toward the head, as you did with the Half-Headstand Posture. Next raise either leg as high as possible and have whoever is helping you grasp it by the ankle. On the count of three, make a little jump, while he or she simultaneously places the raised leg in the corner against the wall. The other leg will follow suit of its own accord. Your assistant can help you hold your legs up by gently placing the hands against them. And that's it! That's all there is to it!

You have managed to stand on your head with both legs straight up, supported on either side by the wall. What you have to do now is relax. If you keep your legs rigid, body tense and spine arched, you will feel so uncomfortable that it would be better to come down immediately. Moreover, if you feel tense, your helper will not be able to raise your legs easily. Consequently, if you find that you remain stiff and tense and can't relax, it is best that you attempt to do the posture at another time.

At the beginning, you should not hold the Headstand for more than ten seconds. Then, slowly lower yourself down, first bending the knees, then lowering the feet all the way to the ground. Remember always to keep the toes inverted; otherwise you may injure them when you reach the floor. If you prefer to have help in coming down—which is not a bad idea until you have completely mastered the technique—bend only one leg, while your helper grasps the other one by the ankle and holds it tightly, letting it follow the one you yourself are lowering.

All this should be done very slowly and gently, without pulling or hurrying or accelerating the natural tempo of your own movements. Of course, your assistant should be standing up to your right if you start coming down with the left leg, and on the other side, if you prefer coming down with the right one.

Once you have come down, remain kneeling a few seconds with the forehead on the floor. Then stand up, raise your arms above your head, take a deep breath and lie down to rest. After a short while take a few more deep breaths.

If you do it this way, the Headstand will be not be difficult at all. There are many people who are able to do it without any previous preparation. Don't forget to point your toes, relax your body, keep your back straight, neck and shoulders free of tension, and elbows not too far apart, as the body's weight must be carried partly by the forearms.

It is so easy to stand on your head in a corner that after some press conferences I often have reporters and photographers successfully trying this posture. Once, after completing a television interview in Washington, I started giving a class in Yoga to a whole room of enthusiastic studio technicians who had been watching the program. Most of them were able to do the Headstand easily.

I must warn you, however, that using a corner to steady yourself has one disadvantage: you can grow so used to doing it this way that it may take you longer to start doing the Headstand without safeguards in the middle of the room. As far as the benefits of the posture go, doing it in a corner or in the middle of the room makes no difference. But if you do want to perform the posture correctly, in the classical way, you should do without any support or help.

TIME: Do the Headstand for ten seconds at the beginning, increasing five more each week. The maximum time for it should not exceed two minutes, if it is done in conjunction with other exercises.

BENEFITS: The Headstand benefits are so numerous that it has been called the "King of Asanas." First of all, it affects four of the most important endocrine glands: the pituitary, the pineal, the thyroid, and the parathyroid, all of which are responsible for our very existence, for they keep the body mechanism in good working order. Consequently, practicing this posture helps to relieve many of our physical and mental troubles, or better still, to prevent them.

Yoga recommends the Headstand especially to those people suffering from nervousness, tension, fatigue, sleeplessness, dullness, fear, poor blood circulation, bad memory, asthma, headaches, congested throat, liver or spleen disorders, female troubles, initial stages of eye or nose troubles and general lack of energy, vitality, or self-confidence. But most important of all is the fact that it affects the pituitary, the gland that controls all functions in our bodies.

There are extremely few cases in which people find difficulties in the beginning. I once had a pupil, a prominent woman on a visit from

New York to California, who was never able to do the Headstand because as soon as she tried it her nose would start bleeding. We let some time go by, and when I saw her again in New York, we tried it again and this time had no trouble doing it. She told me that during that time, she had been practicing other Yoga exercises; she had also been eating one or two slices of raw onion daily. Unable to decide which of the two had been really responsible for her sudden success, we decided to split the credit. I don't think we will ever know the answer to this, and I am simply telling you the story without trying to draw too many conclusions.

CAUTION: The Headstand should not be practiced by people whose blood pressure is either too high (above 150) or too low (below 100). Neither should it be practiced by those who get palpitations while doing it and by those suffering from constipation or when stools are too dry. Likewise, it should never be done by people with pus in their ears, or those suffering from chronic nasal catarrh. Finally, this exercise should be avoided by people with an organically defective pituitary, pineal or thyroid gland, or people who have trouble in their cervical vertebrae or suffer from serious coronary problems.

STRETCHING POSTURE
(Paschimatanasana)

Next we will try the Stretching Posture, called Paschimatanasana in Sanskrit. This too belongs to the group of basic Yoga postures. It closely resembles the Head-to-Knee Posture, except that in this one both legs are stretched instead of just one.

TECHNIQUE: Sit straight with both legs extended, feet together and hands to the sides of the body. Take a deep breath, hold the air for a few seconds while you lift your arms, slightly stretching the upper part of the body; contract your abdomen a little and start exhaling while you slowly bend forward until your hands grasp your big toes or the

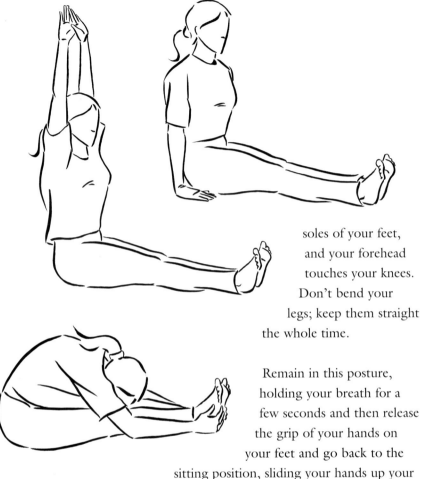

soles of your feet, and your forehead touches your knees. Don't bend your legs; keep them straight the whole time.

Remain in this posture, holding your breath for a few seconds and then release the grip of your hands on your feet and go back to the sitting position, sliding your hands up your legs while you come up. Repeat and relax.

If the posture is not easy for you to accomplish, do the following preparatory exercise: sit straight with legs extended. Flex the right leg and take the top of your foot with the right hand. Inhale and then stretch that leg upward without letting go, while you exhale. Flex your leg again, placing it on the floor. Repeat this movement three times and then do the same with the left leg.

Lastly, flex both legs, taking hold of the toe points of both feet. Inhale deeply and, while exhaling, stretch your legs, sliding them on the floor

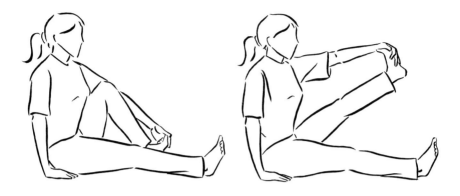

without letting go of your toes and pushing your heels forward. Repeat this movement three times, and you will see how easy it is to do the posture afterward.

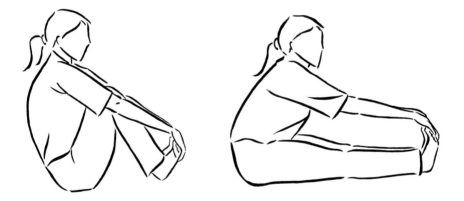

TIME: Remain in this posture from five to fifteen seconds. At the beginning do it twice. If you wish, you may increase the number up to six times, by adding one more every fourteen days.

BENEFITS: The benefits of the Stretching Posture are much the same as those of the Head-to-Knee Posture. It helps to overcome constipation, indigestion and lumbago, apart from reducing abdominal fat. It massages the pelvic region and gives an invigorating pull to the hamstring muscles and sciatic nerves. Through the practice of this Asana, bowels become more active. This posture is also practiced in advanced stages of Yoga for its spiritual values.

CAUTION: When releasing the Stretching Posture and going back to your original position, do it slowly and smoothly, never in sudden, brusque movements. Those who suffer from constipation should practice this exercise with special care. If you cannot reach your feet with your hands at the beginning, hold your ankles or your calves instead; you can also use a belt, a scarf or a towel to pull from, as in the Head-to-Knee posture. Try especially not to bend your knees.

Now lie down and relax briefly.

PLOUGH POSTURE
(Halasana)

Next we will do another of the basic Yoga postures: the Plough Posture. It is called Halasana in Sanskrit.

TECHNIQUE: First assume the Reverse Posture (see p. 99), with or without the aid of a table. Then slowly, without bending the knees, start to lower both legs while exhaling. When your toes reach the floor behind your head, you have achieved the Plough Posture.

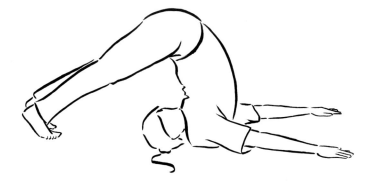

Place the palms on the floor and remain in this position for a while, trying to do deep breathing. This may seem somewhat uncomfortable at first, but it will become easier for you in a few days. Then go back to the original position while exhaling the air, lowering your spine very gently, vertebra by vertebra, until it is completely lying on the floor. In order to do this, bend your knees slightly, place your legs behind your forehead and then, slowly gliding them down over the face, continue slowly until completely resting on the floor.

TIME: At first, remain in this posture for five seconds; then gradually increase the time up to two minutes, adding five seconds every week. Repeat from two to four times, increasing one time every fourteen days.

BENEFITS: The Plough Posture affects the thyroid gland, massages the liver and spleen and stretches the vertebrae, keeping the spine in a youthful, flexible and healthy condition. People who have a tendency to stiffness, obesity, muscular rheumatism, constipation and indigestion, as well as those who have an enlarged liver or spleen, or suffer from arthritis, will especially benefit from this posture.

WARNING: If you have not yet become more flexible through previous exercise, do not attempt right away to practice this posture to perfection, unless you have by nature a very flexible spine. Otherwise, for a few days, try not to touch the floor with your tiptoes. After that, you may try doing it with your head about two feet from the wall, getting into the Reverse Posture and taking the legs back until the toes touch the wall. Then you will start "walking" downwards on the wall.

Take care not to force any movement; instead take small steps lowering your legs as far down as your spine comfortably allows, otherwise you are likely to injure a rigid muscle and the pain may last several weeks. This will frighten you away from attempting the posture again, so please be careful!

For a variation on the Plough Posture, you may bend your legs instead of stretching them; in this case the knees should almost touch the ears and the toes should be on the floor. Once you've finished the posture, lie down, relax and take some deep breaths.

CAMEL POSTURE
(Ustrasana)

Up to now most of the postures you have been learning and practicing require a forward bend; and only one, The Cobra, is practiced bending backwards. The Camel Posture, or Ustrasana in Sanskrit, which you will now do is another backward-bending exercise.

TECHNIQUE: Kneel down, sit on your heels while keeping toes outstretched, and place your hands on your heels. Lean on them and throw your head back if you don't have problems with your cervical vertebrae.

Now, while inhaling deeply, slowly raise the buttocks off the knees, lifting the lower part of the body and arching the spine.

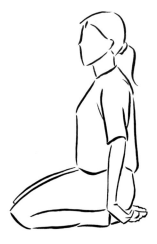
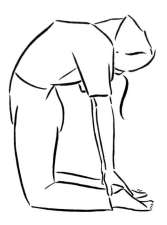

Remain in this posture while you hold your breath; then return to the original position. Sit on your heels, move your head forward and exhale. Rest a while and repeat the whole exercise.

TIME: Hold the posture for five seconds, gradually increasing the time to thirty seconds. Repeat from two to five times. It is better to practice this posture in the morning than in the evening.

BENEFITS: The Camel Posture affects the thyroid glands and the gonads, or sex glands. It gives elasticity to the spine and tones the muscles supporting it. People suffering from gas, constipation, and displacement of the vertebrae and of the pelvic organs—that is, the ureter, urethra, urine bladder, uterus and Fallopian tubes—will greatly benefit from this exercise, provided the displacement is not of a major nature. It is also beneficial for people suffering from kyphosis and asthma.

CAUTION: People suffering from a herniated disk should not attempt this posture, and neither should those with lordosis, scoliosis, or problems in the lumbar region. It is not recommendable either for people who suffer from dizziness or for women during their period. People who have high blood pressure should do it only for a short time.

Those who cannot place their insteps on the floor while doing the posture may place their toes instead and take hold of their heels. This variation on the Camel Posture is easier to achieve.

LION POSTURE
(Simhasana)

Let us now do the Lion Posture, Simhasana in Sanskrit. In spite of its strange and grotesque appearance, this posture has no equal for overcoming various throat ailments, especially tonsillitis and pharyngitis.

One of my students, a lawyer, told me how she once won a case she would otherwise have surely lost, with the help of this posture. On the morning of the trial she awoke with a terrible pharyngitis; she felt desperate. Then, remembering the Lion Posture, she did it about six times in a row. The effect was almost magical—her throat was cured completely. Incidentally, this Asana is exceptional in that it is effective within a few minutes.

TECHNIQUE: Sit down on your heels, or on a chair if sitting on the heels is difficult for you, and place your hands on your knees. After taking a deep breath, stick out your tongue as much as you can, almost to the point of gagging. While doing this, stretch your fingers and separate them, arching them upwards as much as possible. Open your mouth and eyes as wide as you can and tense your neck and throat, as well as the entire body, but especially the throat. Remain in this posture for a few seconds, intensifying the tension; then exhale and relax.

TIME: This posture can usually be repeated two to three times, but if you are on the point of developing tonsillitis or pharyngitis, do it six to ten times in succession several times a day.

BENEFITS: The Lion Posture affects the throat by sending an extra supply of blood to it. It also massages and tones the muscles and ligaments of the throat, at the same time strengthening and invigorating the whole body. People who suffer from enlarged tonsils and a throat susceptible to infection should practice this posture daily.

CAUTION: Do not do this posture immediately after a meal, as you are likely to throw up.

FOOTLIFT POSE
(Ardha Baddha Pada Uttanasana):
Second Movement

We will now attempt the second movement of the Footlift Pose or "Stork," the first part of which we did in Lesson Two; by now you are probably able to remain standing without hopping around on one leg like a lame bird.

TECHNIQUE: Get into the first movement of the posture as directed in Lesson Two. Stand on the right foot, keeping the left foot as high as you can on the right thigh and holding it with the right hand. Keep the left knee at the same level as the right knee. Now take a deep breath and, while exhaling, bend forward until the fingers in your left hand touch the ground. Bend your head down to touch the knee, or try to do so. The left heel should firmly press against the abdomen. Remain in this position, holding your breath; then return to the first position, take a few deep breaths, and relax.

Repeat this exercise and then do the same standing on the left leg. Just as in the second breathing exercise of the First Lesson, keep the buttocks tucked in when bending forward. The bending should be done by the spine from above the waist.

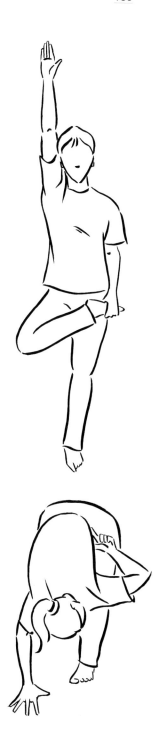

TIME: Hold this position from five to twenty seconds, repeating it two to five times.

BENEFITS: The Footlift strengthens the legs, massages the abdomen and is beneficial for people troubled by constipation, gas, and fat around the waist and in the abdomen. It is particularly good for acquiring steadiness and balance. If you have poor balance, you may do it leaning on the wall.

Breathing Exercises

CLEANSING BREATH

To do the Cleansing Breath, stand straight with feet close together and arms hanging loosely at the sides. Take a deep breath, hold it for a little while, and then purse your lips as if you were going to whistle. Next start to exhale forcefully, but little by little; that is, don't expel the air as if you were blowing out a candle, and do not puff out your cheeks, which should be tight and hollow.

You should do it in successive and forceful exhalations that will feel to you almost like coughing fits that expel the air until the lungs are completely empty. The effort of exhalation should be felt in the chest and in the back.

Rest for a while and repeat. After a week you will be able to repeat this routine several times every day.

BENEFITS: Like its name indicates, the Cleansing Breath cleans and ventilates the lungs, toning the whole body in the process. You should do the Cleansing Breath at the end of each lesson and immediately before the final relaxation.

WALKING BREATHING EXERCISE

Before concluding the lesson with relaxation we will do the Walking Breathing exercise. This is done in exactly the same way as Rhythmic Breathing except that you do it while walking. Each step may be used as a count, as you used the pulse beat in Rhythmic Breathing.

Stand erect, exhale and start walking, right foot first. Take four steps while inhaling and hold your breath while you walk another two; then exhale for another four steps, and take two without air in the lungs. Do not interrupt the walking—keep it rhythmical. The breathing should be continuous: do not inhale in four short breaths, a mistake which many beginners tend to make. Instead, take one deep breath while you count to four, hold it to the count of two, and exhale it to the count of four, holding the emptiness to the count of two. This is the way to complete one round. Make five such rounds a day the first week—no more—adding one round per week.

If you feel that four steps are too long for you, count three steps and hold one. If, on the contrary, four are not enough and you feel you want to continue the inhalation, take six steps or even eight, and hold the breath on a count of three or four steps respectively. In either case, you should take an even number of steps while breathing in and out, and the retention is done in half the time taken for inhalation or exhalation.

You can practice the Walking Breathing exercise not only while doing the corresponding exercises in the lesson, but at any other time while you are walking, especially when the air is pure, as in a park, a forest or at the seashore. You can also do it while you are walking toward your car or going to take a bus or other public transportation, while you climb down stairs, take your mail to the post office, pause for a coffee break in your office, and, in fact, whenever you think of it. Simply stop walking if you are doing so, and inhale and exhale deeply.

After doing this once, start breathing as indicated while you give slow even steps; the important thing is to keep the rhythm.

End the lesson by relaxing and meditating.

Relaxation

Before a new student joins my class, he is generally asked, among other things, what is the reason for taking up Yoga.

The great majority, according to my experience, want to learn how to relax. Even if they have other motives, relaxation is almost consistently among the most important.

Men and women alike seem to suffer widely from what they call "nerves." Constantly you hear them say: "I'm on the edge," "My nerves are in bad shape," "I'm all stressed out . . ."

Such neuromuscular tensions are seldom due to disease of either the nerves or muscles, but rather to reactions of the body to the impressions of the mind. They stem from conscious or unconscious thoughts dictated mostly by different kinds of fears.

Such was the case of a man who came to see me, complaining of nervous tension. "It simply drives me crazy," were his exact words. "The point is that I am in the grip of this thing and can do nothing about it. Take yesterday morning, for instance. I got up feeling fine, completely relaxed. Then came the mail and the moment I saw those bills and the letter from my lawyer I felt my neck muscles tighten; I couldn't stop it. The tension spread to the upper part of my back and shoulders. Then I got a headache and when I arrived at the office I was no good for doing anything. Last night I lay in bed imagining all sorts of strange things, including the loss of my job, and today I feel like jumping into the lake. That tightening of the muscles seems to have no end. Isn't there some way a man can get away from this torment? Loosen up, relax, be himself again?"

It took quite a while to teach this person the technique for deep breathing, for he kept forcing it and therefore did not benefit from it. He seemed unable to relax whenever he wanted to. Finally I made him lie down, close his eyes and imagine he was at the seashore, while the waves rolled in and out, in and out, in and out. Then I knelt behind him so that he could hear me breathe, and I began doing Deep Breathing after instructing him to visualize a wave rolling in with each inhalation, and one rolling out with each exhalation.

"Let me do the deep breathing alone at first," I suggested. "You can join whenever you feel sufficiently relaxed to do so." Within a few minutes we were both breathing in unison.

I have seldom witnessed such a wild outburst of joy as the one this man gave way to following his first relaxation lesson. Once he discovered there was a way to learn how to relax, he was beyond himself with happiness.

In cases like this, the real trouble is that a vicious circle sets up because the person's mental tension is the result of purely physical conditions, while body tension is the result of emotional stresses and strains. Once this circle is closed, it is difficult to break. Thus, for example, when the thyroid is overactive or exhausted as the result of hard living, it may in turn produce a physical state that leads to emotional disturbance; this trouble further accentuates "nervousness" or neuromuscular tension. The more wound up the person is, the harder it is for the body to shake off its stress.

In general terms and limiting oneself to civilized people, the tensions start with their imaginative, fear-ridden responses to their over-complicated environment. The human being's effort to find a way out of this dilemma goes a long way back. He has tried just about every single remedy: alcohol, drugs, cigarettes, long walks, mowing the lawn or playing golf. He tries sex, war, religion and every possible system of evasion. He has even thought to find the solution in death. But his problem is yet to be solved.

In our times the human being has tried escaping toward space. Yet since he can neither run away from nor forget himself, wouldn't the most logical answer be to turn within himself, to search his inner self, and there find the solution to his ongoing troubles? As curious as it seems, this is the only remedy he seldom thinks of trying, except in a few individual cases.

Some years ago, a German magazine carried an article titled, "The Death of the Manager: The Scourge of the Successful Man," where it promoted Yoga, an ancient Indian prescription, as a remedy for the "Manager Disease," encouraging relaxation and daily breathing exercises to do away with tension and prolong life. There was an impressive illustration that pictured the manager lying dead at the entrance to a conference room. A snuffed-out candle in the background stood as a symbol of the premature end of his life, for it could have burned much longer. The silhouette of several Yoga postures below suggested that this was what the manager had failed to do; otherwise he might have prolonged his life.

The article stated that half of the big executives, businessmen, politicians and other people of importance who had recently died "in the prime of life" usually had succumbed to degenerative diseases such as weak hearts or circulatory disturbances. All these men had died of overwork, overstrain, over-exhaustion and over-tension. They had also eaten too much, drunk too much, and smoked too much. But their main trouble had been stress. Therefore diabetes, arthritis, coronary thrombosis, constipation, headaches, neurasthenia, obesity and a hunched back had been common ailments among them. Usually they had tried to fight their troubles with pills and drugs, which did not touch the real hidden enemies—fear, tension, and the wrong idea of what living really is.

"The manager," this same article went on, "could have smoked cigars and sipped drinks another thirty years had he known about Hatha Yoga." After this statement a description of the breathing exercises and postures followed, urging everyone to learn from Yoga its amazing technique for relaxing the mind and body, for preserving youth and health, and for prolonging the span of life.

Except for the cigars and drinks, which to me are a strange kind of reward to expect for taking up Yoga, the article was much to the point and very convincing. Furthermore, it probably aroused great interest in Yoga among those who read it. For why not get to know the secrets of relaxation, youth, health and longevity, by learning the lessons from those who have proven through the centuries the effectiveness of their system, instead of relying on panaceas offered by people who themselves are engaged in a "rat-race"?

It is true that no machine or mechanical trick, no pill or prescription, can be effective for very long when the problem is to relieve the mind from stress and the body from strain. Physical and mental relaxation is one of the fundamental main beliefs of Yoga. You yourself may have noticed by now, if you have been doing the relaxation exercises regularly at the end of every lesson without skipping any, how these exercises result in muscular agility and mental ease. This will become still more apparent as you practice the Headstand, which we began today. Still another step toward true relaxation will come with the meditation, which will be part of your final lesson.

Yet the reader may well wonder how the Headstand can relax you, when, on your first attempt, it made you feel anything but comfortable. The answer is simply that you should not become impatient—it will not be long before you will feel at ease while standing upside down. There is a good physical explanation for this, and I would like to go into the physiology of what happens when the human body is upturned this way.

The Endocrine Glands

The Headstand Posture has an effect on two of the glands we have already described as the most vital ones in our body: the pituitary and the pineal, both of which are located in the head. When you stand on your head, a large amount of blood—blood that is being further enriched through deep breathing—flows to the head, carrying an extra supply of energy to these glands.

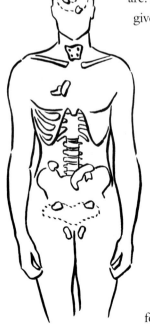

You may remember from the chapter on the endocrine system in my previous book *Forever Young, Forever Healthy* what the functions of the different glands are. If not, the illustration on this page will help give you an idea. As you see, the endocrines are all situated at strategic points in the body. In addition to the pituitary and pineal in the cranium, the thyroid and parathyroid are behind the larynx at the base of the neck, the thymus is in the upper part of the chest above the heart (incidentally, this gland shrinks in size and importance as we stop growing), the two adrenals are on top of the kidneys, and the gonads, or sex glands, lie in the lower part of the trunk below the digestive organs.

The functions of all the endocrine glands are interconnected, although each has a different function to perform. Another name for them is glands of internal secretions, because they secrete various hormones without which our organism could not function properly. Hormones are best defined as those various substances formed inside the endocrine glands that activate specifically receptive organs. Thyroxin, for instance, is a hormone secreted by the thyroid gland, cortisone by the adrenal glands, and so on. If any of the endocrine glands become either over- or underactive, we may lose or gain weight in various parts of the body, or suffer from different disruptions.

The main gland, or, as it has often been referred to, the "boss of them all," is the pituitary, for it regulates the activities of all the others. Although very small in size—no larger than a pea—it is of paramount importance to our well-being. As many as twelve various hormones are known to be manufactured inside it.

"We know, for example," writes Dr. John A. Schindler in his provocative book, *How to Live 365 Days a Year*,[1] "that there is one hormone of the pituitary that raises blood pressure, another that makes smooth muscles contract, one that inhibits the kidneys from producing urine, one that stimulates the kidneys to make more urine. Then there is a whole group of hormones that regulate the other endocrine glands of the body. These other glands produce many more hormones to regulate just about everything that goes on in our bodies."

The reason I am giving the reader all this information in this discussion is so that you may understand, more or less, many of your health problems. Think of the human body as if it were potentially threatened by an enemy army, whether in the form of bacterial invasion, virus infection, or emotional stress. The aftereffects of drugs, accidents, operations, exposure to high altitude, excessive heat, cold, moisture or dryness, muscular overexertion, nervous breakdowns, and even starvation are included among these dangers. Think of the pituitary gland as the chief who alone must fight off any attack by any of these enemies, and you will begin to get the picture.

More specifically, the various dangers threatening our well-being are sometimes referred to as stressors, while the result of their negative influence is called stress. This is the way Dr. Hans Selye describes them in his monumental work, *Stress of Life,* and in *The Story of the Adaptation Syndrome.* He explains that the most dangerous and most powerful of all stressors are those of our own emotions when they worry and upset us. That is why the job of an executive often carries with it diabetes or peptic ulcers: it is the result of having to deal with all kind of unpleasant duties, the duties of a hard fighter. A man in a subordinate job, on the other hand, is more likely to suffer from colds, tiredness, nausea, weakness, arthritis, asthma, inflammation and all sorts of aches and pains. This is, of course, a generalization: anyone may be afflicted by ulcers or arthritis.

The findings of Dr. Hans Selye have thrown a completely new light on the functions of the pituitary gland and its capacity to mobilize the body's defense forces against any kind of invaders.

It is impossible here to go into further details on this fascinating subject, as it requires more time and space than I have at my disposal. But I do wish to warn the reader that most of our illnesses are not due to the toxins, to the virus or bacteria as such, but to the stressors that, offsetting the normal activity of the pituitary gland, throw it off balance, and thus lower our resistance to illness.

Because the worst offenders are the psychic stressors that produce emotional upsets, a high-strung, intellectual person is more subject to them than a less sensitive individual. And what we often blame on our nerves should actually be blamed on our glands.

Here is a secret of relaxation and youth given by a man who doesn't know what tension and stress are and who, at ninety-four, looks, feels and works like a person half his age. "My strength lies in never hating or even opposing anyone," Jacques Romano told the writer interviewing him. Then he explained that he was a Buddhist when with a Buddhist, a Christian when with a Christian, a dog when with a dog, etc. To sum up it up, he said, "Treat people as if they were flowers and you will have a happy life."

You will probably now see for yourself where Yoga comes into the picture. The practice of the Headstand has a direct influence on the functions of the pituitary gland that regulates our entire well-being. Rhythmic breathing and relaxation exercises enable us to overcome muscular and mental tension, which also adversely affect the hormonal secretion of this gland.

Thus you can see how Yoga can restore the normal working order of our entire organism and understand why the relaxation of the body and mind go hand-in-hand with health, youth, happiness and a long life.

1. Englewood Cliffs, N.J.: Prentice-Hall, Inc., 1954.

Lesson Four • Fourth Week

Physical pain, melancholy, unsteady limbs,
irregular inhalation and exhalation,
all are causing distraction of the mind.

—YOGA DARSHANA

Today you are starting on the second half of the course; in only three more weeks you will have completed it.

So far, you have learned seven of the basic Asanas, ten additional postures, and six breathing exercises. Choose from among them those that best suit your particular physical condition as well as your personal needs, ability and time. From now on, use them as the basis for your own daily exercise routine. Continue with the basic postures and vary only the additional ones. On the first day of each new lesson you may, if you wish, give preference to the new postures, in order to get acquainted with them.

Even after you have completed the course, it is advisable for you to reread the instructions once in a while before assuming one posture or another, since there is always a tendency, of which you are unaware, to start deviating from the correct way of doing the exercises.

In order to perfectly assume the postures, the instructions should be carefully reviewed, as there are always details that were overlooked at the beginning.

I remember once watching one of my first students doing the postures together with his wife and children. The four of them went through the exercises at such high speed, and keeping such perfect timing between each other, that it looked to me more like an acrobatic performance than a Yoga lesson. For without good posture, concentration, relaxation, and, above all, deep breathing, these postures cease to be Yoga Asanas, no matter how well executed they are, and become ordinary calisthenics. This is the sort of mistake you will avoid if you check your practice according to the instructions given.

Yoga postures should remain an individual experience at all times, regardless of the number of people who are executing them together.

Today, after you have finished the Rocking exercise, we will start our lesson with the Headstand, which we will do against a wall, but only if you feel absolutely sure that you can do it this way. Otherwise, continue as before, using the corner to lean on until you no longer need it.

HEADSTAND
(Shirshasana): Second Stage

TECHNIQUE: To do the Headstand against the wall, you should place a mat about a foot from the wall. Then kneel down in front of it, interlock your fingers, and place the hands on the mat. The distance between the hands and the wall should be approximately that of the length of your arm from your wrist to your elbow.

Place your head with weight on a spot about an inch above the forehead on the mat, and nestle it in the hollow of the palms, finding a comfortable position. When you stand on your head, always remember

to lean on the forearms for better support and balance. Now move your feet
closer to your head, take a deep breath,
and, lowering your buttocks, take a quick
jump or do a similar movement to get your feet
off the floor.

Continue to raise your bent legs very slowly.
When you are halfway up, tuck your buttocks in
and don't straighten your legs yet, as otherwise
you are bound to lose your balance and fall
over. To avoid this, quickly bend your
knees and prop up the soles of the feet
against the wall as seen in the picture.
Remain in this position for a while—your
body in a straight line from head to knees, legs
bent, soles of feet on the wall for support. Now, keeping your feet
together, close your eyes and do deep breathing.

After a while, straighten your legs and try to separate your feet from
the wall, contracting the buttocks to keep balance. Hold this position
for about thirty seconds, then bend the legs and start lowering them
slowly until the toes touch the floor. Don't forget to keep the toes
inverted so as not to injure them. It is very important that you descend
slowly, otherwise you may fall on your knees and hurt yourself.

If you feel you are losing your balance while standing on your head,
quickly put your feet against the wall. But do not remain leaning
against the wall with your legs outstretched, as this will result in the
arching of the spine and it will be harder to accomplish the perfect
posture. You should bend the legs, and, when you feel confident
enough, separate them from the wall and straighten them to achieve
the final posture.

Once you have reached the floor with your feet, raise your arms, take a deep breath and lie down to rest and relax.

TIME: Start by remaining ten seconds in the Headstand. Increase the duration of the Headstand by five seconds each week. The maximum time is two minutes, when done with other exercises.

CAUTION: Keep in mind the same advice given for the Headstand's first movement in Lesson Three.

SWAN POSTURE
(Swanasana)

Next we will do a posture that, as they say, kills two birds with one stone. The first movement affects the spine, shoulders, pelvic area and wrists, while the second one benefits the digestive organs, abdomen and knees. The starting position is the same as in the Cobra Pose (see p. 69).

TECHNIQUE: Lie down on your abdomen with your palms on the floor at shoulder level, elbows up and toes stretched. Take a deep breath and, leaning on the palms, raise your head, shoulders, and torso, separating the abdomen from the floor until you have straightened your elbows completely.

As I said, this posture resembles the Cobra Pose, with the difference that here the elbows are kept completely straight. Remain in this position for as long as you feel comfortable, resuming normal breathing. Don't raise the palms of your hands up; they should remain flat on the floor.

To come back, first inhale and, while exhaling, take your buttocks back to your heels and rest there, pressing the abdomen against the thighs and touching the forehead to the floor, as you see in the picture.

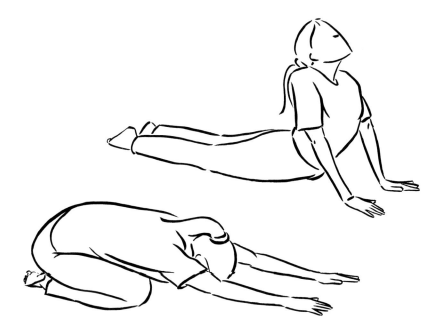

Remain in the same posture for a while, holding your breath. Then start exhaling, while you raise your buttocks off your heels and move your body forward, without changing the position of your palms, until you are back to the previous Cobra-like posture, but with arms completely stretched. Remain in this posture, holding your breath; then, as you exhale, move back into the kneeling posture again.

TIME: Repeat this to-and-fro movement three to four times, making sure you do the breathing correctly.

BENEFITS: This exercise strengthens the spine, arms, wrists, chest and throat. It also straightens the back and shoulders. While in the kneeling position, the thighs massage the abdomen by pressing against it and the shoulders and arms get a good stretch. The to-and-fro movements help promote a better intestinal evacuation and reduce fat.

CAUTION: People who have trouble in their lumbar vertebrae, those with a herniated disk, high blood pressure or serious coronary problems should refrain from doing this posture.

TWIST POSTURE

(Matsyendrasana): First Movement

Rest a while before starting this posture. It is
called Matsyendrasana in Sanskrit, which
sounds like a tongue twister for most people
who are not Indians, and is also quite a spinal
twist for everyone. We shall do it in three
stages so that it is not too
difficult for you to learn.

This posture also belongs
to the group of basic
Yoga postures.

TECHNIQUE: Sit up straight with both legs outstretched. Cross
your right foot over the left knee, place it firmly on the floor, keeping
the left hand on the instep of the right foot. Be sure that the right
ankle is stuck close to the left knee. Stretch out the right arm and,
carrying it toward the right and backwards, twist it as much as possible around the back of your waist line. Your right hand palm should
be opened toward the outside and the wrist should be resting on the
left hipbone. Keep both
head and spine straight,
and the entire sole of
your right foot on the
floor. Inhale deeply
and, while exhaling,
slowly turn your head,
shoulders and waist
toward the right as
much as you can. When
you have finished exhal-
ing all the air, you will
notice that you are able to

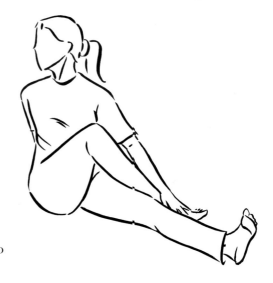

twist a little more to the right. Do not bend your head while doing so, and keep your chin up.

Remain in this position, holding your breath for as long as you can; then start exhaling, while slowly unwinding the twist until the head, shoulders and back are in the original position again. Pause for a while and repeat the Twist. Then reverse the position of legs and hands, and assume the same position with the twist to the left side.

TIME: Maintain this posture for five seconds, holding your breath. Increase the time up to one minute, adding five seconds every week. When holding the posture for more than several seconds, resume deep breathing while remaining in the posture, but always unwind on exhalation. Repeat the twist two to three times.

BENEFITS: The Twist affects the adrenal glands. It also tones up the kidneys and relieves a congested liver or spleen. The effects of constipation and indigestion are offset by the practice of this posture. The spine and its deep muscles become strong and flexible; stooping shoulders, a bent back and bad posture are also corrected. People suffering from asthma should emphasize this posture as well as the Shoulderstand, the Headstand, and the Supine Posture.

The Twist, especially the last stage of it, is a wonderful posture. When you begin to slowly turn around your body, you should imagine yourself like a peacock majestically unfolding its large, colorful fan.

After finishing this exercise, lie down and rest until your breathing is back to normal; then breathe deeply several times.

ABDOMINAL LIFT

(Uddhiyana Bandha)

Now we will practice the Abdominal Lift, called Uddhiyana Bandha in Sanskrit. It is considered one of the very essential Yoga exercises and should be practiced not only for its physical values but also for the way it also influences our psychological growth. This last is true even though this pose does not strike either a particularly aesthetic or impressive figure.

TECHNIQUE: Stand with feet about a foot apart, inhale deeply and exhale forcefully. Then, without inhaling again, draw in the abdominal muscles with a strong upward pull until a hollow forms under the ribs.

Place your hands on your thighs, bend the knees a little, and slightly tip your trunk forward without lowering it. The diaphragm will then rise easily. Press your thighs firmly with your hands by leaning on them. Stay in this position as long as you can without breathing. Relax. Stand up straight and resume normal breathing. Repeat the Abdominal Lift only once more. Do not breathe at all while doing it.

TIME: This exercise should not be done more than twice in the first few days. You can gradually bring it up to seven times, adding one time per week.

BENEFITS: The Abdominal Lift tones the abdominal muscles and stomach, relieving, also, discomfort from gas, constipation, indigestion and liver trouble. Yogis also practice this exercise to develop spiritual strength. It is considered the best exercise for toning up those nerves that have their roots in the solar plexus region. It also regulates the functioning of the sexual and suprarenal glands.

The Abdominal Lift is also often used by the yogis for interior purification. In order to accomplish this state, drink several glasses of water, always at room temperature, with one-fourth teaspoon of salt per glass, and then do the contracting and relaxing movement several times in standing, sitting and lying positions.

As a matter of interest, I should mention here that one of my students sent me a booklet on the "avalanche treatment," which is based on cleansing the intestine by drinking large quantities of salt water and afterwards assuming five different positions in each of which successive contraction and relaxation of the abdomen is practiced. This is just another example of how, whether knowingly or not, Yoga methods have been gaining access into Occidental health practices.

CAUTION: The Abdominal Lift should not be practiced by people suffering from a weak heart, high blood pressure, or serious abdominal or circulatory troubles.

To be able to check on whether the abdomen is being pulled in properly, do this exercise in front of a mirror placed against the back of a chair or sofa. Tip the mirror a little; otherwise you will not be able to see much, since your trunk must bend slightly forward. Be careful not to bend the knees too much, however, as the body should not be lowered, but merely be slightly inclined.

To begin with, it may be easier for you to practice a variation of this Bandha. Instead of keeping your abdomen drawn in, pull in and let go, repeating two or three times in quick successive movements. Relax and stand up straight. Repeat once again and make sure that after the pulling-in movement, which should be done with full strength, you do not use any force at all for the pushing-out movement: this pressure should be gentle and it happens when you relax the abdominal muscles. In other words, the accent is on the sucking-in movement, not on the letting go.

After having practiced this exercise for three days, you can do this quick contracting and relaxing exercise first, then follow with the full Abdominal Lift, which you should keep up for as long as you can without breathing.

CHURNING POSE
(Nauli)

The Churning Pose, called Nauli in Sanskrit, should not be attempted until after you have gained full mastery of the Abdominal Lift.

TECHNIQUE: Assume the Abdominal Lift as described above, but place your hands a little farther up and point the fingers toward the inside of the thigh. While holding the air in, try to isolate the recti muscles[1] by pushing back with an effort and a contraction that is similar to that used when one feels constipated, the difference being that the "push" should be directed to either right, left or middle rectus in order to isolate it. If you have succeeded in isolating the middle rectus, it will stand out like a rigid vertical band, because in this area above the pubic bone the recti muscles alone can be separated. After having isolated the medium rectus, proceed in similar manner to separate the right, then the left rectus.

When isolating the right rectus slightly incline the body to the right; and when working on the one to the left, incline yourself to the left. To make it easier to practice this exercise, place a mirror on a chair, as recommended for the Abdominal Lift. When you have succeeded in isolating each in turn, begin to "churn" these three muscles from left to right or from right to left, whichever is easier for you.

It is not so easy to obtain immediate results from this exercise, for which you have to be patient. Often people push all the abdomen out or do not perform the contraction properly. If you find yourself doing either, you can avoid this mistake by relaxing the muscles immediately and starting all over again. Keep trying until you succeed in separating the recti muscles. Do not overtire yourself by making too many attempts at one time.

BENEFITS: The Nauli Pose tones up the abdominal region and keeps it healthy. It is also a good exercise for people troubled by indigestion, constipation or malfunction of the liver, spleen, kidneys, and pancreas. It helps as well to overcome ovarian insufficiency and painful periods.

CAUTION: People over forty-five should not start on the Nauli exercise without consulting a specialist first. The same applies to those who suffer from appendicitis, intestinal tuberculosis or high blood pressure. Children should not practice this exercise before the age of puberty.

FOOTLIFT POSE

(Ardha Baddha Pada Uttanasana): Third Movement

TECHNIQUE: Stand straight, place your right foot high up on your left thigh, holding it up with your left hand while putting your right arm around the back of your waistline, as

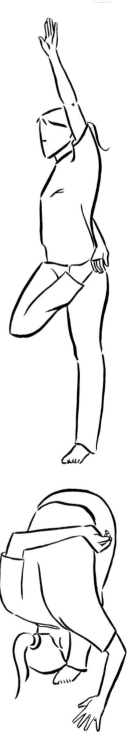

you have done in the twist. Now with your right hand grasp the toes of your right foot while letting go with the left hand and, inhaling, taking it up as shown in the picture. Exhale while standing straight. Do one deep inhalation and, while exhaling, bend forward, until you touch the ground with your left hand, and, if possible, bring the forehead closer to the left knee. The right heel should firmly press the abdomen. Try contracting your buttocks.

The third and final stage of the Footlift Pose may present some difficulties at first. Therefore it is meant only for more advanced students.

TIME: Maintain this posture for a few seconds, then return to the original standing position. Reverse position of your hands and feet and repeat the Footlift or "Stork" standing on your right foot.

I suggest going back to this posture's benefits in Lesson Three, when I described the Second Movement.

Breathing Exercises

FIRST BREATHING EXERCISE

Stand erect, feet together. Inhale deeply while slowly raising your heels off the floor until you are standing on your toes. Remain in this position for a few seconds, holding your breath. Exhale while at the same time slowly lowering your heels to the floor. Repeat two or three times.

Now do the same, getting up on the toes of your right foot while keeping your left foot "hooked" behind the right calf just above the ankles.

TIME: Do this exercise two or three times, then repeat after reversing legs.

BENEFITS: If you practice this exercise you will acquire good corporal balance. It also strengthens your ankles and develops your calves. It is a good exercise for fallen arches and flabby calves.

SECOND BREATHING EXERCISE

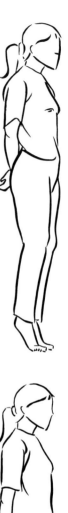

Stand straight, feet together, hands at both sides of your body. Inhale deeply while raising your arms, without bending them, above your head until the palms of both hands join each other. Stay in this position holding your breath for a few seconds; then turn palms over so that the back of your hands are touching, and start to exhale slowly while lowering outstretched arms. If you do this exercise correctly, you will experience a tingling sensation in your palms and fingers.

As you hold your breath with the palms of your hands joined above your head, you should lock your throat by tightening its muscles to make sure that no breath escapes.

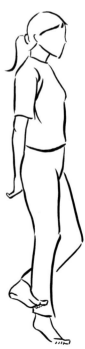

Repeat this exercise after a short pause, and finish with the Cleansing Breath.

This breathing exercise should be practiced immediately before the relaxation moment.

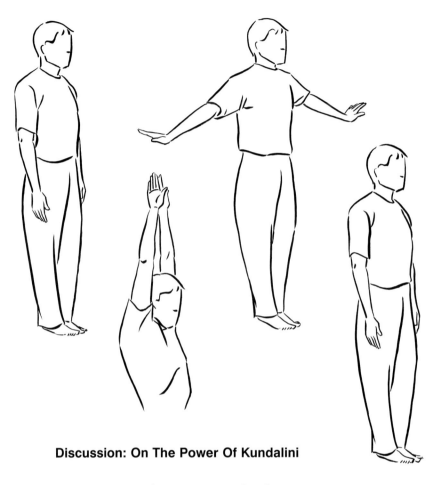

Discussion: On The Power Of Kundalini

*Man can send a current only along
a wire, but nature needs no
wires to send her tremendous energies.*

—SWAMI VIVEKANANDA

The subject of our discussion today is the most secret and sacred of all Yoga practices: the awakening of the mysterious Kundalini, or Serpent power.

This practice belongs to the very advanced stages of Yoga, and it would be both impossible and dangerous to attempt to accomplish it here in the Western hemisphere. The truth is it cannot be done by means of written instructions alone as each step requires the close supervision of a guru or spiritual guide.

But as a student of Yoga, you should have at least a theoretical knowledge of Kundalini since its awakening is at the heart and root of Yoga.

You will undoubtedly recall that at the end of the First Lesson of this book I mentioned the word Prana, and explained that this is an energy that exists in fluidic form in the atmosphere and is present in everything that lives, from amoeba to man. The air, sunshine, water, plants, minerals, food—all are impregnated with this life substance, which is the source of all energy, vitality, and power.

The yogis teach that Prana circulates in our bodies through a network of special channels that they have named nadis, from the word "nad," meaning "movement" in Sanskrit. The nadis are distributed throughout our astral body, just as the arteries, veins and all nerves run through our physical body. The astral body is supposedly the same shape and size as the physical one, but of a finer substance. It is not visible, except to a clairvoyant. The yogis ascertain that we possess seven bodies, including our gross physical body. Being astral and not physical matter, these bodies are not visible to the naked eye. It was the ancient yogis' clairvoyant capacities that made their research work and findings possible: otherwise how could they have made such accurate studies of the human organism with all of its functions thousands of years before there were any instruments available? Clearly they must have known about the existence of the endocrine glands, since most of the Yoga postures were devised in order to affect one or several of these glands. Modern science, on the other hand, knew next to nothing about them until 1899, when endocrinology was officially born.

However, Western scientists took, and continue taking, a very skeptical attitude toward the whole Yoga theory of Prana, for they can find no instruments that register it. Hence, they dismiss the entire subject as nonexistent.

Incidentally, the existence of Prana was known not only to the yogis of India, but also to the ancient occult schools of the Egyptians, the Hebrews, the Tibetans, the Chinese, later the Japanese, and finally the Greeks. Even the early Christians knew of this mysterious cosmic energy, for which there were many different names.

In the book of Genesis, for instance, the Hebrews called it Neshemet Ruach Hayim, which means Breath and Spirit of Life. The Tibetan Naldjorpas and the Japanese Zen school, which originated in China where it was brought by the Hindu missionaries, included Pranayama, the Yoga breath-control exercises, in some of their practices: it was designed to increase the circulation of Prana in the body. To keep the nadis clean, the yogis have devised special purification processes called Shodana.

The three most important nadis are the Shushumna, the Ida (pronounced Eeda), and the Pingala. Shushumna is the chief nadi, located inside the spinal cord, with Ida and Pingala spiraling on either side like the two snakes in the caduceus of Mercury.

Shushumna is represented by the straight rod; Ida and Pingala by the intercircling snakes, and the two petals of the Ajna chakra by a pair of wings. The small sphere on top of the rod supposedly symbolizes the pineal gland.

Ida, flowing through the left nostril, is lunar, feminine, and cooling; Pingala, flowing through the right, is solar, masculine, and heating.

The physical counterparts of Ida and Pingala are probably the sympathetic chains of our nervous system, while that of Shushumna is the spinal cord.

Before we go any further, I suggest that you take a look at the chakra illustration on page 167 to get a clearer understanding of this subject.

In the picture you can see the seven major centers of Cosmic Energy situated on the spinal cord, or Shushumna nadi, and intertwined by the other two nadis, Ida and Pingala. These centers are called chakras, wheels, or padmas, lotuses. They are the astral counterparts of the plexuses of our anatomy. However, they should not be identified with them because, just like the nadis, the chakras also belong to another dimension.

The Location of the Chakras

There are seven important chakras of major significance. The lowest, Muladhara chakra, is situated at the base of the spine. It controls the process of elimination and corresponds to the sacral plexus. This is the real occult center of the body because it encloses the secret, dormant energy called Kundalini, which is symbolized by a snake coiled three and a half times with its tail in its mouth. It closes the entrance to the chief nadi, Shushumna, which takes its root in the Muladhara chakra. Incidentally, all of Asia, as well as ancient Egypt and Greece, frequently represent Divine energy in the form of a snake.

The second is the Swadisthana chakra, situated opposite the genital organs. It controls sexual desires and corresponds to the epigastric plexus.

Third is the Manipura chakra, which is opposite the navel and is concerned with digestive functions. Its counterpart is the solar plexus.

The fourth, or Anahata chakra, is at the level of the heart. It controls respiration and corresponds to the cardiac plexus.

The fifth, the Vishuaddha chakra, behind the throat, controls speech and corresponds to the pharyngeal plexus.

The sixth is the Ajna chakra, located between the eyebrows. It controls the autonomous nervous system and corresponds to the cavernous plexus, or more probably the pineal gland. It is the seat of the mystical "third eye" of Shiva, the seat of clairvoyance, according to the yogis. The biblical Yehovah is also often represented as having it. The Ajna chakra is where Shushumna, Ida, and Pingala come together and form the sacred knot called Triveni.

The seventh and last chakra is the Sahasrara, corresponding to the cortical layer in the brain. It is also known as the Thousand-Petalled Lotus.

All the lotuses, or chakras, have a certain number of petals that range from two to sixteen; the highest chakra is represented as having a great number of petals.

When the power of Kundalini is awakened by special exercises, it passes from the lowest chakra, the Muladhara, through the central nadi, Shushumna, and through all the other chakras, which begin to "spin" like true wheels and open their petals like lotuses. When Kundalini finally enters the last and highest center, the Sahasrara chakra, the yogi reaches his goal: the divine marriage between Spirit and Matter takes place. At this point, his individual consciousness unites with Universal Consciousness, and he enters a state of ultimate bliss, called Samadhi. It must be noted that even among the yogis, there are very few among them who truly reach a complete state of spiritual illumination.

Great mystics and saints of all religions have also on occasion experienced and described this state but without possessing the knowledge of how to awaken it consciously.

The ascending of the power awakened in Kundalini, achieved by various practices and exercises, is the most secret of all Yoga teachings and is always verbally transmitted from master to disciple. It cannot and should not be put into writing.

In his *Higher Psychical Development,* Howard Carrington says that much has been done in order to prove that the mystical "Tree of Life" mentioned in Genesis is connected with Kundalini. This extraordinary energy that brings with it the knowledge of good and evil was wrongly awakened by a being known in the Bible as Adam. The author suggests that the entire Genesis legend of the serpent is, according to the Oriental point of view, a way of symbolizing the awakening of the fire serpent Kundalini, which is also the primordial electrical energy known as Speirema, or the serpent coil.

In the sacred writing of India this energy or power is spoken of as "the slumbering serpent." In the book of Genesis it is symbolized as "the serpent, more subtle than any beast of the field which the Lord has made." When this force started stirring within Eve, she felt tempted to misuse it.

Directed downward to the lower physical centers, the serpent force brings knowledge of evil; directed upward, to the brain, it brings knowledge of good. Hence the dual operating of the solar force that is symbolized as the "Tree of Knowledge of Good and Evil." This key energy, fundamental in our bodies, is closely connected with the fundamental sex energy and may be controlled and transmuted by certain Yoga practices.

As to the subject of sex itself: Like so many others, you may probably be under the wrong impression that Yoga promotes and advocates the suppression of sex, since many yogis try to lead an ascetic life. Let me tell you here that this is not so. The yogis merely know the secret of transmuting sex energy into more subtle forces, called ojas, and directing these into psychic channels. Through this transmutation, excess sex energy is neither lost nor suppressed: it is merely changed into finer substances, just as ice may be changed into water, or water into steam.

Suppression of sex usually results in all kinds of mental and physical troubles, in abnormalities and perversions. Now then, this same energy, instead of being utilized in the normal manner or in healthy exercises and mental activity, may be drawn upward to the solar plexus or to the brain. This is a Yoga practice. When I described it in the chapter on sex in my book *Forever Healthy, Forever Young,* I only very briefly mentioned that sex energy was closely connected with the Kundalini power, but did not touch upon its actual operation. Let us now take a closer look at it.

When awakened in a yogi, this solar energy gives him stability, harmony, freedom from desire and a lasting feeling of happiness. He then arrives at the realization of the true Self. The divine spark in him grows into a flame and merges into the Universal Consciousness. This realization of God—or whatever you wish to call It—is the final goal of all yogis. It is the highest state to which a human being may arrive on this Earth.

Many need a lifetime, or several lifetimes, to achieve this state, while for others it may only take a few years. It may also come suddenly, like an unexpected gift. This has been known to happen not only to yogis and rishis of India, but to mystics, saints and spiritually developed persons the world over.

We ordinary human beings cannot expect to reach this exalted state of consciousness as long as we lead a worldly life and are caught in the web of its illusions. But it is good to know that a paradise-like state can exist even on earth, that it is a reality, and that we too, eventually, in other lives to come, may enter this realm of eternal bliss and ineffable happiness.

To quote from *Yoga* by Major General Fuller, "The Yoga philosophy has been the solace of millions for many centuries not only in India but throughout the world. This philosophy has produced the greatest and most influential masters, Gautama, Christ, Mohammed, whose mastery over the Unknowable has been the driving force of nations. All these men were yogis of one sort or another. Their lives, though outwardly differing from one another were inwardly the same, and so was their teaching, which, in each case, led the aspirant to the one Reality, the Peace which passeth understanding."

1. The recti muscles are any of several straight muscles in the abdomen.

Lesson Five • Fifth Week

*The numerable forms of philosophy, of arguments,
and of the rules capture the intellect in their nets
and lead it away from the true knowledge.*

—YOGABIJA UPANISHAD

HEADSTAND
(Shirshasana): Third Stage

We shall begin this week's lesson practicing the final stage of the
Headstand. In case you are wondering why we always start with this
posture, which should be only preceded by the Rocking, the reason is
that it is easier to keep your balance standing on the head when the
body is not yet tired from other exercises. This time let us try the
Headstand in the middle of the room, without the support of walls.
Choose a room that is big enough for you to stand on your head freely,
because chances are you will have to restart this posture many times.

TECHNIQUE: First place a pillow or a big cushion next to the mat
on the floor; kneel down in front of it and put your head down the

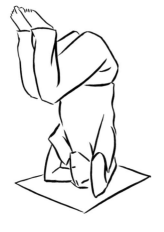

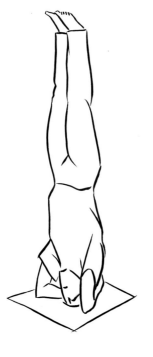

way you have been doing up to now. Lift your legs by straightening your knees and holding yourself up on the toes of your feet; take one or two steps toward your head. Take a deep breath and, with a gentle jump, bend the knees, bringing them close to your chest, and lift your feet off the floor. Slowly start raising your legs while keeping the knees still bent.

Just before straightening the legs, contract your buttocks, as it will help you keep your balance. Also remember to keep the elbows not too far apart as the whole body is supported not only by the head, but also by the forearms. Now straighten your legs.

Don't be afraid if at the beginning you end up falling when you least expect to on the other side of the pillow or cushion; you should keep on trying and practicing until you are able to maintain your balance. This may take several days, but do not get impatient and under no circumstances try to get up on the head more than four or five times at one time, as it is an exhausting exercise. After having done your best in four or five attempts, lie down to rest even if you have not been successful. Do not push things too far.

Once on your head, keep your spine and legs straight; your feet and body should be relaxed. Do deep breathing with your eyes closed. Remain in this upside-down position for a few seconds. To come back down, bend your knees, bringing your heels close to your buttocks; then bring forward both legs in a flexed position, trying to touch your chest with the thighs. Next straighten your legs until your feet touch the floor. Don't forget to keep your toes stretched. Stand up slowly, stretch both arms above your head, take a deep breath and lie down to rest.

Don't ever remain standing on your head if you are not feeling comfortable. Bring your legs down and relax. I cannot emphasize enough that the head, neck, shoulders and spine should be relaxed. If you find yourself unable to overcome the fear of getting into an upside-down position, it is wise to continue with the Half-Headstand until you feel you are inwardly ready to try the complete posture. Don't feign the braveness of someone jumping into the deep end of a swimming pool, because you will become even more tense and fail. You should try accomplishing this posture when you feel relaxed and self-confident, without any sense of fear, impatience or belligerence; otherwise stand on your head in the corner or near the wall. Enjoy it—never force the issue.

As we have already seen the benefits and warnings concerning the Headstand in a previous lesson (see p. 127), please look them up to be sure that you make no mistakes.

TIME: Remain in this posture for ten seconds at first, adding five more per week. If you practice the Headstand alone without any other exercise preceding or following it, it can eventually last five minutes if practiced by an advanced student; otherwise the limit is two minutes.

TRIANGLE POSE
(Upavishta Konasana)

After taking a little rest, get ready for the Triangle Pose, or Upavishta Konasana in Sanskrit.

TECHNIQUE: Sit up straight and open your legs as wide as possible.

Inhale deeply and while exhaling stretch out your arms and bend forward to the right until you can take hold of the toes of your right foot with both hands. Touch the knee of that same leg with your forehead. Remain in this position while holding your breath; return to the original position and inhale. Repeat the same movement, bending toward the left and then forward.

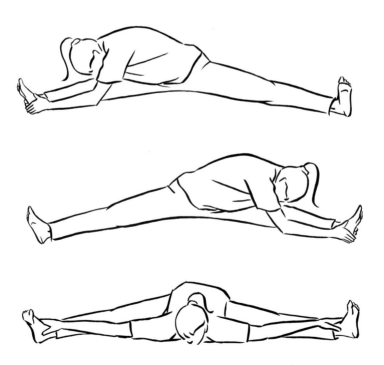

Now extend both arms to the sides while starting to exhale and at the same time bend your body forward until you can, with each hand, grab the toes of the foot of that same side, while you touch the floor with your forehead. If you cannot reach down that far, bring your head down as low as you can. Take hold of your feet with belts or straps if you can't reach the toes.

TIME: To start with, keep this posture as long as you can hold your breath. Later on increase its duration to one minute, during which time you will do deep breathing. Repeat two or three times.

TWIST POSTURE
(Matsyendrasana): Second Movement

Now we will practice the second movement of the Twist Posture. I hope it does not present any difficulties after you have been practicing the easy version of it for a whole week.

TECHNIQUE: Start by assuming the first movement of this Asana, which should be familiar: First stretch out both legs, crossing the right foot over the left knee. Now bend the left knee so that the left heel touches the right buttock. Place the left hand on the right foot as you did before, and wind the right arm around the back of the waistline, with your hand open and your palm facing outward. Take a deep breath and, while exhaling, slowly make a complete turn to the right, keeping the shoulders straight and the chin up: first the head, then the shoulders, then the back, from the first to the last vertebra.

TIME: Remain in this posture for ten seconds holding your breath and then inhale; exhaling, straighten your back, shoulders and finally your head, coming back to the original position. Repeat the whole exercise once and then reverse the position of the legs and arms and repeat the twisting movement to the left.

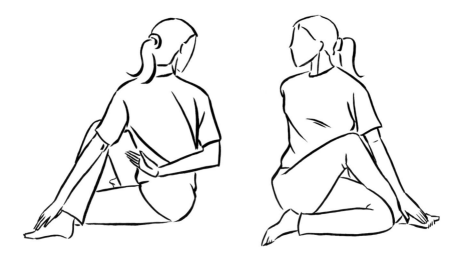

After you finish doing this posture, lie down on the floor and rest. When your breathing is back to normal, take a few deep breaths.

SHOULDER STAND
(Sarvangasana)

Now we will practice the Shoulder Stand, called Sarvangasana in Sanskrit. Following the Headstand, this posture is considered one of the most important Asanas. You will see it practiced in many gyms and health clubs, but it is seldom coupled with the deep breathing, without which it is no longer a Yoga posture but an ordinary exercise with much less therapeutic value. It has been called "The Candle" because the body is kept as straight as a candle in this posture.

It is a very important Asana for both men and women. Should you imagine that you are "too old" to try it, just look at the daily example of groups of older people in our classes, some of them more than eighty years old.

You will find it very similar to the Reverse Posture, with the difference that the body is kept in one straight line from shoulders to toes and the position of the hands is changed from the hips to the spine for better support. Moreover, the Reverse Posture affects mainly the gonads or sex glands, and, partially, the thyroid, while the Shoulder Stand affects the thyroid more and gonads less.

TECHNIQUE: Lie down on your back and start inhaling deeply while you slowly raise your legs until the toes point to the ceiling. Support the back of your spine with both hands, letting the body rest on the nape, neck and shoulders. Keep it as straight as a candle. Press the chin against the chest and straighten the knees. Close your eyes and breathe deeply, trying to remain steady in this position.

Remain like this for a few seconds; then, while exhaling, slowly go back to the lying position: first, bend the legs, place the palms of the hands on the floor, and then, curving the spine, start gradually to unfold yourself as if you were a rug, until your entire back touches the floor. Straighten your legs, inhale deeply, and, exhaling, lower yourself as slowly as you can.

TIME: Remain in the Shoulder Stand posture ten seconds, gradually increasing five seconds every week. If this is the only posture you are practicing, without any other exercises to precede or follow it, it can be retained for five whole minutes by an advanced student.

BENEFITS: The Shoulder Stand affects the thyroid gland and the sex glands and has, therefore, a powerful influence on the entire organism. It vitalizes the nerves, purifies the blood and promotes good circulation. It strengthens the lower organs and helps them to stay in place preventing their displacement or prolapse. It is especially recommended for women after childbirth. People troubled by asthma, constipation or indigestion should diligently practice this posture. It is also helpful in reducing painful menstruation, other female disorders or ailments, and seminal weakness.

CAUTION: The Shoulder Stand should not be practiced by persons with organic disorders of the thyroid gland, and if the person has chronic nasal catarrh, it should be done with caution. Neither should it be practiced by people with cervical troubles, high blood pressure, or nasal congestion. Women should abstain from doing it during their period. When there are serious spine problems it may be replaced by Viparita Karani Mudra, as I teach it in Lesson Two (see p. 99).

SUPINE PELVIC POSE
(Supta Vajrasana)

If the Shoulder Stand is done for a long time it produces a feeling of discomfort in the neck; you should therefore always follow it by the Supine Pose to relax the neck.

TECHNIQUE: Kneel down with knees kept together and feet apart, resting the insteps on the floor. Sit down between the heels, placing the buttocks on the floor and the palms of hands on the thighs—you shouldn't sit on the heels. Close your eyes and slowly deep breathe.

In order to go on, you should feel well relaxed in this posture. Next, start reclining the body backwards, leaning first the elbow and forearm of the right arm, then the elbow and forearm of the left, until the whole back is lying on the mat. Put your hands behind the nape of the neck. Don't arch your spine, which should be as flat as possible. Close your eyes and deep breathe.

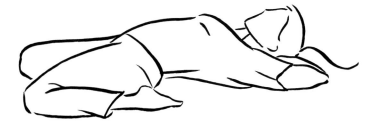

Go back to the Pelvic Posture, leaning first on the elbows, then on the forearms, and, finally, on the palms of the hands. Rest a while before starting the breathing exercises.

TIME: You should remain in this posture for five seconds, increasing it by five seconds a week until reaching a maximum of two minutes. Relax and rest.

BENEFITS: This posture exercises a healthy influence on the suprarenal glands. It limbers and stretches the neck, strengthens and tones the nervous system, the kidneys, the stomach and the intestines, the pelvic organs and the nerves connected with the sex functions. It also benefits the solar and sacral plexus; prevents muscle, nerve and joint stiffness; exercises a healthy rub on the lumbar area, relaxes the nervous system and soothes the mind.

Breathing Exercises

RECHARGING BREATH

Now stand up, keeping the feet close together and hold your hands near the chest, with palms joined, thumbs placed on the sternum and the rest of the fingers oriented upwards. Close your eyes and take several rhythmic breaths, visualizing how with every inhalation you draw in the vital cosmic energy, or Prana, and with every exhalation you send it circulating all over the body. A receptive mental attitude on your part greatly contributes in the absorption of Prana from the air. And by keeping your hands and feet together, the Prana will not "leak out," since you have closed the circuit, so to speak.

Another variation of this exercise is done sitting in the Lotus Pose with palms on the upturned soles of your feet.

This exercise helps restore vitality when you feel depleted of all strength and energy. You can also use the Recharging Breath for protecting yourself from the influences of disturbing vibrations. For this purpose it will suffice to keep the thumb and index finger together, as if you were holding an invisible flower in each hand; then do the rhythmic breathing and at the same time visualize that you are building a protective circle around yourself.

In India this kind of breathing is often done when taking long trips on trains with people whose vibrations might be of a low or evil order. A friend of mine, a well-known artist in California, used to practice this kind of breathing when he used the New York subways or public buses because he was extraordinarily sensitive to other people's vibrations, to the point that they would make him feel sick and dizzy.

WOOD-CHOPPING MOVEMENT

Stand with your feet wide apart, stretch your arms out, clasp your hands, interlocking the fingers, and imagine yourself holding an axe. Inhale deeply, slowly raising your hands above your head and taking them stretched far back, flexing your body as much as you can. Remember that you are lifting a very heavy axe. Hold your breath for a moment, then, vigorously exhaling through the mouth, swing the axe forward with a powerful motion as if you were actually trying to chop wood. But instead of going back to the standing position, after having done the first wood-chopping movement, relax and let your arms hang totally limp for a few seconds.

Repeat this exercise several times, always imagining that you are really chopping wood. The arms and spine should be in the same line; don't move your buttocks when bending down. All the movement should be done from the waist upward, arching your spine.

This exercise is energizing and strengthening; it's also good for keeping the spine flexible and for reducing abdominal fat.

CAUTION: Persons with a weak heart and women suffering from female disorders should do this exercise very gently.

As always, finish the lesson with relaxation.

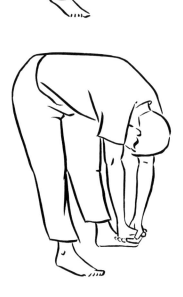

Discussion: On the Yama-Niyama and Contemplation

*The way of the spirit is selflessness; the way
of the body is selfishness. It is up to us
to establish the balance between the two.*

—SIGFRID KNAUER, M.D.

In India, before a Yoga aspirant is ready to begin his training he must
accept, at least for the period of his discipleship, the Yama and
Niyama, which are the ten rules of the Yoga code or morals.

Yama consists of the following precepts:
1) inoffensiveness (non-destructiveness, non-injuriousness);
2) truthfulness;
3) non-stealing;
4) non-desire for what belongs to others;
5) continence (frugality, indifference toward sexual enjoyment).

Niyama instruct:
1) purification (internal and external cleanliness);
2) contentment;
3) strength of character (abstinence, austerity, forbearance, discipline,
non-complaint, patience, calmness of mind);
4) study;
5) complete self-surrender to the Lord (which includes sharing with
others that which has been given to you).

Certainly these precepts may sound familiar to you. Do they not
remind you of the Beatitudes and of the Ten Commandments?

But how many commandments and beatitudes do you still remember?
Are you aware of your attitude toward them? Do you actually try to
follow them? Or are you indifferent to them?

Many people, for example, sincerely believe they are not guilty of killing. But if they were to compare their reaction to the commandment, "Thou shalt not kill," with the attitude of, say, Albert Schweitzer, they would be forced to change their position. For Schweitzer did not allow any kind of killing in his jungle hospital in Equatorial Africa where he preached "reverence for life"—not only human life but all life.

I was reminded of this when I heard J. Allen Boone, who wrote *Kinship with All Life,* telling us about the time when, just as he was about to spray his room in order to rid himself of ants, it suddenly occurred to him that they too were part of the Great Life and had a right to exist. After some hesitation he decided to talk to them, telling them that he respected their desire to live and would not kill them, yet since their proper place was outside in the garden, would they please leave. He gave them two days' "notice," warning them that he might not have another choice but to use the poison if they refused to listen. "Believe it or not," he said in conclusion, "within two days the ants had actually disappeared."

This amusing story made a big impression on me. Soon after this, Olga, our maid, discovered a stream of ants in the corner of the living room where a big night moth lay dead behind the curtains. Remembering Allen Boone's experience, I asked her not to touch them, but to let me handle them. After she was gone I sat down on my knees to present my plight to the ants, asking them to go where they belonged and ending with a promise to keep some sugar for them outside. A few days later they were gone. "Because there is nothing to attract them," argued Olga; but when she lifted the curtain, we saw two more big moths lying on the floor and not a single ant around. Overwhelmed with joy, I looked at her triumphantly.

This small incident opened up a vast new world for me. I know there are yogis who, because they are attuned to every living creature, can tame even tigers and other wild animals; but since I don't think of an ant as an animal, and I am not a yogini, I experienced a feeling of true happiness when my gentle persuasion worked. From then on I started talking to all sorts of creeping and crawling things, which included a beautiful snake I encountered in the ruins of an ancient temple in Cambodia.

Of course I am not so sure that I would be as successful with a tiger or a wild boar. Therefore I had better change the subject and return to Yama, which we were discussing.

I suggest you write down on a piece of paper the ten Yamas and Niyamas, or the Ten Commandments, or the Buddhist Commandments, which are also ten in number. Here they are:

1) Do not kill, but respect life.

2) Do not steal or rob; but help everybody to be the owner of the fruits of his labor.

3) Abstain from impurity, and lead a life of chastity.

4) Do not lie; be truthful. Speak the truth with discretion, fearlessly and with a loving heart.

5) Do not invent evil sayings, nor repeat them. Do not criticize, but look for the good in your neighbor, so that you can defend him with sincerity against his enemies.

6) Do not swear, but speak decently and with dignity.

7) Do not waste your time with gossip; follow your purpose or keep silence.

8) Do not covet or envy anything; rejoice at the good fortune of others.

9) Clean your heart of malice and don't cherish hatred, not even against your enemies; embrace all living beings with kindness.

10) Free your mind of ignorance and be anxious to learn the truth, especially in the one thing that is needed, in case you fall prey to either skepticism or errors.

I suggest that every night you take up just one point to meditate on. Don't be in a hurry to answer it. Ponder about it and take time to carefully think about its meaning before going on to the next one.

A student of mine once cheerfully subscribed to the first Niyama, thinking that by brushing her teeth and taking a daily shower she was obeying the precept of internal and external cleanliness. She had to reconsider, however, when it came to keeping the colon clean, and furthermore to cleansing the mind and heart of hatred, envy, jealousy, anger, malice, greed, and lust.

The last Yama concerns the sex life of the disciple, or chela. It is necessary, as you already know after having discussed the power of Kundalini, to keep sexual energy so that it may be converted into finer energies, or Ojas. Yoga does not advocate the suppression of sex, but a sublimation of it. Remember, too, that all the strict rules and Yoga disciplines concern only a true disciple, not a student of Yoga such as you.

But generally speaking, the Yama-Niyama, or the Commandments, should also be taken into account by all human beings, especially by those interested in spiritual advancement and understanding.

To recognize and understand our shortcomings, and to see ourselves in a true and objective light is a most difficult thing, much more difficult than to do your hair, to shave, or to put on makeup and dress for a performance without a mirror. That is why we need an impartial third person, such as a teacher, to point out our faults to us. We cannot possibly see ourselves nor trust completely the criticism of our family or friends since, as is so often the case, they can all be prejudiced in one way or another.

What should one do if there is no one to turn to for advice and guidance, no one to point out our wrongs to us and to tell us the truth about ourselves?

When I once found myself in such a situation—I felt completely alone and was surrounded by people to whom Yoga was nothing more than a target for jokes and cruel remarks—I remembered the advice once given me by Krishnamurti[1] in a desperate moment of my life, when I was going through very painful and distressing personal experiences.

"Do you know the real cause of your suffering?" Krishnamurti asked me then. "It is fear, although you may not realize it. You are unhappy because you are afraid to face your troubles and are trying to patch them up somehow. You want to run away from them instead of calmly examining what has caused your sorrow. You must face utter loneliness. If you really want to free yourself from the cause of your sorrow, you must be alone, and in facing that loneliness you will become watchful and alert. One is fully aware only when one is not trying to avoid something, nor trying to escape from the inevitable, which means to be alone. Through the ecstasy of that solitude you will realize the Truth."

Krishnamurti was right. When I began to analyze my problem, fear was at the bottom of my troubled state of mind. According to Krishnaji it was necessary to adopt an objective point of view, to see things from a different angle. But how was I to go about it? He advised me to remain completely alone and to see no one for several days. "Stay with your problem and look at it very closely. When you do that you will not be afraid of it any longer."

I followed his advice although I could not see how it was going to help me. Until then I had always thought that sympathy and warmth would help me more than solitude. I was wrong. After a few days spent alone in tears and despair, a wonderful feeling of peace and joy suddenly entered my heart and filled my entire being. It seemed that all my torments belonged to a remote past and had stopped meaning anything to me.

Later, when I recalled the change this experience had brought about in me, I resolved to keep regular days of complete silence so that I might turn for advice and inspiration to that most reliable friend, teacher, and guide—the Supreme Self, the Truth within us. Setting aside a special day for this "meeting," I decided also to fast on the day of silence, to see no one and speak to no one, in short, to remain "absent" from everybody and everything.

In the beginning it felt a little strange to remain alone in my room in a sort of vacuum all day long. I made it a point not to go on with my usual routine but to spend the day meditating, listening to music and chants, reading the poems of Krishnamurti, books on Yoga and on the lives of great sages and saints. At times, I would just let my thoughts pass by like the white clouds outside my window.

Soon after the beginning of the meditation I would become acutely aware of a presence that would fill the room like the blue smoke of incense. At first I would remain motionless, overwhelmed with joy at the visit of my unseen guest who soon became my judge, advisor and friend, one with whom I could frankly discuss all my troubles, difficulties, and shortcomings.

It is not difficult to solve a problem once you can see things from the detached point of view of an onlooker who is fully aware of the real, objective motives underlying every action. No cheating, no concealing, no twisting of facts is possible. One's most secret and hidden thoughts are brought to light and one's actions stand before one in all their nakedness. One knows then what is right and what is wrong, the reasons for having done this or the other thing, and what has brought about someone else's reactions.

Towards the end of the day I would generally break the silence and the fast. Sometimes I kept it till the next morning, reluctant to leave that different world I had discovered. That day of silence, which I kept once a month, became a powerful source of energy and inspiration to me during one of the most difficult periods of my life.

Once, when coming down from my bedroom to take a walk around the garden, I happened to overhear our house boy answer the telephone by saying: "Yes, Missi home, only she not talk, not eat today." Since he was Chinese, he did not approve of this.

From time to time all of us should make a point of clearing our mental storeroom in case it becomes overcrowded with fears, unsolved problems, worrisome thoughts, suppressed emotions and thwarted hopes. We would undoubtedly be much better off if we did so. Usually we keep all this bottled up until finally something explodes either in the form of a nervous breakdown, a serious illness, or a violent rebellion of one kind or another.

Unfortunately, there are few people who are capable of facing the whole truth, because there is always a part that seems to get lost the moment one tries to put thoughts into words, whether because of fear or of shame at exposing one's whole self to another person. But when you turn in all earnestness to the Higher Power within you, no pretense is needed any longer.

If you find it impossible to arrange for a whole day of silence, try to spend a quiet half hour alone at the end of every evening and let all your day's activities pass one by one before the Supreme Judge within you—together with the thoughts, feelings and motives that went into each one of them. Don't cover up or pretend to hide anything. Do not justify yourself nor apologize for your motives; above all, do not try to blame someone else for what has happened: make an honest effort to find out what your mistakes are and where lies the motive for them.

"I don't need to keep any special hour for silence," a woman once said to me, "since I live alone and have no one to talk to anyway." She had missed the whole point, of course, for one can actually remain alone for hours and days on end with the most trivial, superficial, and senseless thoughts, jumping from one to another like a grasshopper. If the hours of solitude are not used for introspection, contemplation and meditation, they have no special value and most likely will become an empty, monotonous time.

A quiet afternoon of deep reflection may allow you to look deep down in your "inner chamber," where you will see yourself as you really are, and thus recognize your faults and solve your problems. We know so little about ourselves!

I know a woman, for instance, whose cousin was so talkative that no one could stand her in the family. When she was told about the problem, she felt so hurt she refused to believe it, because she thought of herself as a quiet person who seldom opened her mouth. Finally someone had the bright idea of recording her conversations and then playing them back to her. The effect was startling. The poor woman was completely disheartened, because up to then she had not realized that she talked nonstop.

Self-discipline is not as hard as one sometimes imagines and may even turn into an interesting experiment. We know of instant metamorphoses of sinners into saints, but in most cases we have to make a constant effort to remain alert. "Know thyself." Difficult? Yes, but it certainly is worth trying.

Now one last bit of advice: When reflecting upon your day's actions, thoughts, and words, dwell more on your shortcomings than on your accomplishments. For accomplishments will present themselves naturally and spontaneously to you, and you may run the risk of complimenting yourself for every little thing, like that young Boy Scout who, while putting down his good deeds for the day, wrote proudly: "Got a chair for Grandmother!"

1. Krishnamurti, reverently called Krishnaji in India, is widely known as a thinker, writer, and speaker. Among other works, he is the author of *Education and the Significance of Life, The First and Last Freedom,* and *Commentaries on Living.*

Lesson Six • Sixth Week

*Concentration is the source of strength
in politics, in war, in trade, in short in all
the management of human affairs.*

—RALPH WALDO EMERSON

You are now starting on the final week of our Yoga course. You have learned a great deal in this short time and I hope you have derived some benefits from what you have learned. Now you must pursue the daily practice of the Yoga postures, without growing sluggish just because you have completed the lessons.

It is usually a good idea to do the exercises with a group at least once or twice a week. This allows you to share your knowledge with others and also to continue perfecting yourself.

After finishing the course, you will have to decide on a schedule for your daily practice, selecting those postures you will do every day, and those you will leave for occasional practice.

Keep in mind that the most important are the ten basic Asanas: the Headstand, Shoulderstand, Reverse Posture, Plough Posture, Supine Pelvic Pose, Yoga Mudra, Lotus Pose, Stretching Posture, Twist Posture, and Cobra Pose. You have learned them all in the past six weeks and you should keep them up. The other postures can be varied according to your needs, time availability and preference. Each person has his or her own favorite postures. Some prefer the Cobra, others the Twist or Reverse Posture. The Headstand is a favorite with a great many people.

For you, the average Occidental with so many other things to do in the course of the day, the basic ten Asanas, two or three breathing exercises and a few extra postures performed occasionally will be enough to keep you in a healthy and youthful condition.

In India, the yogis usually favor about eighty-four Asanas, thirty-two of which are considered very beneficial, and ten are actually essential for the well-being of every individual. The original number of Yoga postures described in the old texts reached eighty-four thousand, but I doubt that there is a single yogi today who knows them all.

Practice Schedule

Here is the order I suggest for your exercise schedule, unless you prefer some arrangement of your own that might be more suitable to your particular needs.

We are not counting the leg-stretching exercise you are to do in bed before getting up. We shall begin with the Rocking exercise, the one you are supposed to do first of all, immediately after getting up. Next, go on to the Headstand, which should never be omitted under normal circumstances, as it is the most beneficial of all postures. I myself managed to do it on a long airplane trip, performing it while everyone else was sleeping so as not to attract attention. My teacher, Sri Krishnamacharya, used to say one should stand on the head whenever one felt tired, hungry, worried or sleepless. This, by the way, is not senseless advice. On the one hand, the Headstand can actually put you to sleep when, for any number of reasons, you are suffering from insomnia; on the other hand, it tones and energizes the body when you feel tired or low.

After the Headstand, you should perform the Shoulderstand, followed or preceded by the Reverse Posture. You may alternate the two, practicing the Shoulderstand one day and the Reverse Posture the next. Then comes the Plough Posture, which should be followed by the Supine Pelvic Pose. This last posture will relieve any tension in the neck that might have been produced by the Shoulderstand and the Plough, which is the reason for putting it in here. If you are familiar with the Fish Posture from my previous book, you may alternate it with the Supine Pelvic Pose.

Next do the Yoga Mudra. If you are not yet able to assume the Lotus Pose, practice the Knee Bouncing exercise first. Follow this with the Stretching Pose. Next practice the Twist, the Cobra, and finally the Abdominal Lift.

Now you can go on to the practice of any other Asanas for which you have the time and inclination.

Do not forget to rest between the exercises. Give more time to those postures that, according to your experience, are more beneficial to you, even if they do not belong to the group of basic Asanas. Always finish with a few of the breathing exercises and the Relaxation.

ANGULAR REST POSE
(Supta Konasana)

Now let us try something new: the Angular Rest Pose, or Supta Konasana in Sanskrit.

TECHNIQUE: Lie down on the floor face up and adopt the Plough Posture; then separate the legs as far apart as possible, stretching them well. Take hold of the big toe of both feet, by inserting the index and third fingers between the big and second toes.

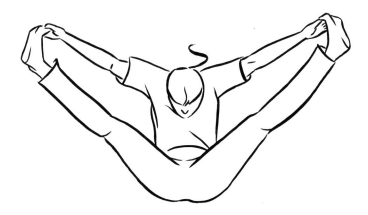

TIME: Start holding this position for about five seconds and breathe deeply. Then bring your feet together again, take both arms to the sides of the body, and start to straighten the spine very slowly in order to return to the original position. Rest a while.

BENEFITS: The Angular Rest Pose combines the benefits of both the Shoulderstand and the Plough Posture. It is also a good exercise for acquiring a sense of balance.

ANGULAR BALANCE POSE
(Urdhva Konasana)

TECHNIQUE: Sit up straight with knees bent, making both feet touch at the soles. Hook index and middle fingers around the big toes as you did in the previous posture. Take a deep breath, and,

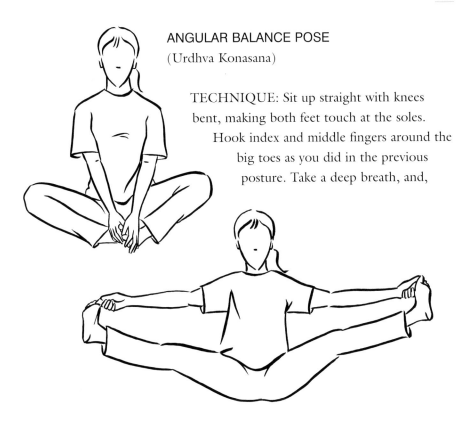

while exhaling, lift your feet off the ground and start stretching your legs sideways very slowly until both legs and arms are completely straight. Do not slant the body, which should rest balanced on the inferior part of the spine or coccyx.

Start keeping this posture for about five seconds, breathing deeply. Then, still holding on to your toes, take your body back until you find yourself in the Angular Rest Position once more.

TIME: In the beginning, remain in this posture for about five seconds, trying not to lose your balance. Repeat several times, changing over from one position to the other and back without letting go of the toes.

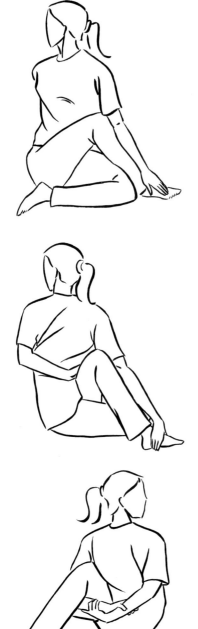

At first you will find it difficult to hold yourself steady in both these postures, for as soon as you assume the sitting position, you will feel pulled back and tend to fall, whereas when trying to get into the Angular Rest Position you will feel pulled up again. In order to keep your body balanced in this pose, pick out a specific point on the floor or in front of you, and gaze at it steadily.

TWIST POSTURE

(Matsyendrasana): Third Movement

The third and last movement of the Twist Posture is done almost like the second, only here you change the position of the outstretched arm.

First, get into the second posture or movement of the Twist, as given in Lesson Five: bend the left leg, place the right foot next to the opposite knee, the left hand on the toes of the right foot, and the right arm on the back of the waistline.

Now raise the left arm, place the elbow on the right knee and glide it down along the right side of the thigh until you can reach the ankle of the right leg with your left hand.

Next, assume the Twist Pose while inhaling deeply; then exhale and twist your shoulders back and your head to the right.

Repeat the process two or three times, change the position of the legs and arms and repeat the Twist to the left.

The Twist gives many beginners a lot of trouble at first. I remember that slender six-foot young man, a hero of many adventure movies, who asked in the middle of my class:

"Are my arms too short or am I too fat?" Neither was the case, of course. What happened was his limbs were too stiff and his spine not flexible enough to accomplish this posture.

"But I will manage getting into this posture, even if I break my arms and back trying to do so," he announced, while watching his wife and children do it with the greatest ease. He was eventually able to do it, without the slightest damage to himself. But it took time.

Breathing Exercises

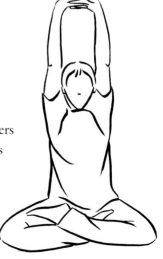

FIRST BREATHING EXERCISE
The Mountain Pose (Tadasana)

Assume the Lotus Pose or sit with your legs crossed. Raise your arms, interlock your fingers and then twist your hands so that your palms face the ceiling. Stretch your arms. Do deep breathing while remaining in this posture.

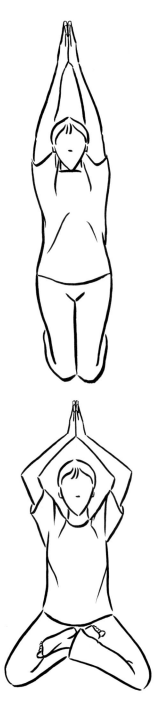

Here is another variation to the same one: kneel down, keeping your body straight from the knees up; stretch your arms up above your head, keeping them straight with the palms joined together; do deep breathing in this position.

There is a third variation that is quite difficult, so you should not feel discouraged if you don't manage to hold this position. First, assume the Lotus Pose; then, raise your buttocks off the floor and balance the body on the knees. The arms should extend above the head, palms together without interlocking the fingers. It is very important to stretch the arms without losing stability while you do deep breathing.

This posture and all its variations are called The Mountain Pose, or Tadasana in Sanskrit.

SECOND BREATHING EXERCISE

Stand up facing the wall. Stretch your arms forward, leaving a space of a few inches between your fingertips and the wall. Then, keeping your whole body stiff as a board, place both palms on the wall with your arms stretched and elbows straight: this will make your body tip slightly forward. Take a deep breath. Then slowly exhale while you bend your arms until the top of your forehead reaches the wall. Keep the soles of your feet completely flat on the floor while you do this. Now inhale again while you stretch your arms and push your body away from the wall. Exhale while you bend your arms. Repeat this movement back and forth several times.

Always remember to keep your body completely straight. The normal tendency is to bend the waist a little, but with this you ruin the effect of the exercise. Your only movement should be that of alternately bending and straightening your arms.

After a few days you may try to do this exercise faster. Do it as follows:

Take a deep breath and, while holding it, do several of these push-up movements; then exhale. Rest, then repeat. This exercise reduces fat in the forearms and ankles, and makes them stronger. It also develops the chest and firms the muscles of the bust, forearms, and calves.

Still more effective, but more difficult, is the exercise described when practiced on the floor instead of against the wall; but after practicing this exercise against the wall for some time, you may do it on the floor without falling on your abdomen.

Lie down on your stomach, with the tip of your toes on the floor and your palms on the ground at shoulder level. Take a deep breath and, while holding it in, stretch and bend your arms alternately, keeping

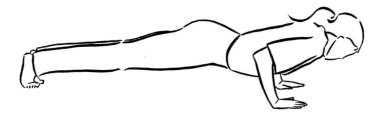

your body stiff and motionless. Then, while exhaling, lower yourself slowly to the ground, so that first the chin and chest descend, and then the abdomen. Don't forget to concentrate on correct breathing.

Finish the lesson with the Relaxation.

Discussion: On Concentration and Meditation

When the mind has become poised,
the Self appears in its true state and we do
not have to make any effort to perceive it.

—SWAMI PARAMANANDA,
Concentration and Meditation

The topic we will discuss to conclude our course will be concentration and meditation, for these form an essential part of the training of a Yoga student.

What is the basic difference between concentration and meditation? Concentration involves the mind, while meditation occupies the heart and the individual's whole being.

"Concentration," to quote Patanjali's *Yoga Aphorisms,* "is holding the mind steadily fixed on some particular object. Meditation is a continuous flow of thought on that object." In concentration you stay "on this side" of the particular object, whereas in meditation you go beyond the limits of earthly manifestations. The source of meditation is always of a spiritual nature, whether it is a Christian, a Buddhist, a Hindu, a Jew, a Moslem, one who belongs to some other religion or none at all.

The ability to concentrate is the mark of genius; the ability to meditate is the mark of saintliness.

Degrees of depth of concentration and meditation naturally vary with the individual. There are people who cannot remain without being distracted for more than a few seconds at a time, whereas others can stay concentrated on one thing for hours on end; this depends on the natural aptitude of the individual, as well as on the practice and training he or she has had. Unfortunately, the art of concentration is seldom practiced in the Western world, where everything is done to constantly distract the mind, which eventually ends up completely dissipating itself. When our mind is excessively overburdened with too many superficial and unimportant ideas it finally loses the ability to concentrate, discern, and discriminate.

As a result there are a greater number of people who never form the habit of thinking their own thoughts, making their own decisions, and solving their own problems. They grow into emotionally immature men and women who are unable to draw upon their own inner resources and who become completely dependent upon what other people do, say or think. Like small children, they begin to look for external diversions, something to excite them and break the monotony of their empty and meaningless existence.

Our mind is almost the only source of our pleasure and pain, failure and success, well-being and disease. This is true of our physical illnesses as well. It is said that almost all our diseases are psychosomatic in origin. This means, actually, that the illnesses have originated in the mind, whether by fear, worry, anger, jealousy or other hostile emotions.

This does not imply that the disease, a consequence of those mental and emotional states of mind, is not completely real. Symptoms may often be treated therapeutically, yet any radical cure can only be effected through the mind, since that is the seat of the basic causes of the disorder.

It seems strange, but many people, especially men, resent being told that their illness is due to emotional stress. "Ridiculous," snapped one businessman who came to see me. "If I can't sleep, it's just on account of this damned herpes, and my doctor told me that Yoga-breathing and relaxation might help. But I'm not a hysterical person. I'm a sound businessman and a very successful one at that!"

However, when I talked with him, I discovered he was not nearly as invulnerable as he thought he was. He admitted that he had been overworking of late, that business wasn't as good as it used to be, that he felt tired at times, and that a misunderstanding he had with a brother, who was also his business partner, had hurt him deeply. When we finally discovered that his herpes had appeared for the first time the day after he had argued with his brother, I managed to convince him to have an honest talk with his brother, although at first he would not hear of it. As I expected, the businessman's troubles vanished when his mind was put at ease, and he not only was able to sleep soundly again but got rid of the herpes as well.

Sometimes the mind behaves like a mischievous monkey that will play all sorts of tricks on us unless we watch it carefully. To illustrate, let us go and watch Mr. John Brown as he prepares to have breakfast after a disturbing and restless night. We come upon him as he searches for the belt to his jacket. He is getting more annoyed by the minute. Finally, he gives up on his search and goes down to the garden to have his coffee. To his surprise, he sees his belt lying in the grass under his bedroom window. Pleased and happy to have found at last what he was looking for, he starts to pick it up when his wife cries, "It's a snake, be careful!" Stepping back quickly, he collides with the maid who drops the breakfast tray. The hot coffee spills not only over the new jacket but also on Mr. Brown's little son who has come over on his tricycle to see the snake, and who now starts crying miserably when he feels the pain of the burn. At last the gardener, alerted by all the commotion, arrives with a big shovel to kill the snake. He stops and grins broadly. "That's no snake! That's the old garden hose I threw away this morning." And that is what it actually was all the time. So you see, Mr. Brown was imagining things when he exclaimed: "There's my belt!" and when he was told: "It's a snake!" But the consequences of his mind-tricks were very real and tangible: his little boy is covered with blisters, the china is broken to pieces, the new jacket is stained and the morning is ruined for everybody.

Who is to be held responsible for all this? Mr. Brown? His son? The gardener? The maid? His wife? They will probably accuse the maid for running into Mr. Brown with the tray, but the real culprit of everything—Mr. Brown's mind—will escape free of blame.

Yet if Mr. Brown's mind had remained calm and objective in the first place, he would not have been so easily irritated, nor would he have excited himself or become frightened. Neither would his imagination have so quickly turned the old hose first into a belt and then into a snake.

If we knew how to concentrate and make good use of our minds, our lives would often be very different. We would not only be free of our daily fears, but would also make a success of almost everything we chose to do, whether in the field of art, science, business, politics, or personal relations.

He who has mastered the art of concentration usually develops a magnetic, vibrant, and inspiring personality to which people are easily drawn.

Take the biography of any successful individual and you will find that even if he or she started their career without money or education, they always possessed one important quality, namely the ability to concentrate. Without this quality they would have never been a success.

Concentration may even be taught to a child through games as soon as he begins to think independently, at the age of about six or seven. I recall one such game we used to play in my family. It was a guessing game. One of us would pretend we had been given a certain sum of money with which to buy whatever we pleased, except that it must be neither black nor white in color. We were also not allowed to answer "yes" or "no" to the questions the others asked while trying to guess what we had bought. It took a lot of concentration for a child not to say "yes" when asked whether she liked the dress that she had bought, or refrain from saying "no" when questioned whether it wasn't a white one.

There are dozens of games like this one that may be played with children and with adults together, provided the grown-ups are not too busy, too lazy or too disinterested.

Interesting experiments with thought-projection have been conducted in Los Angeles, where I wrote this book, by a prayer group formed by Franklin Loehr, who showed us some astounding results produced by the influence of concentration on plants. He had, for instance, a large pot covered by lush greenery on one side, while the other half was completely barren—just plain earth. We were told that an equal amount of seeds had been planted on both sides of the container and that both sides had been given exactly the same attention, with only one exception: the group had been praying regularly for the seeds on the right side to grow and live and for those on the left side to wither and die.

The question of whether it is right to pray for the destruction of any life, even plant life, is another matter, and one we will not discuss here. Nor will we discuss the fact that during a war both sides pray regularly for the victory of their own armies and the destruction of the enemy!

The power of positive thinking undoubtedly works. But so does the power of negative thinking. Like electricity, power itself is neither positive nor negative; it simply exists, and it is up to us to put it to use one way or another. That is why in Yoga, concentration is usually preceded by the Yama-Niyama and followed by meditation. Both, it is felt, help the student avoid possible abuse of his or her thought-power.

In most people the driving force behind concentration is usually desire. When a person desires something passionately, he or she automatically concentrates upon it and is driven towards the achievement of his or her goal. The goal itself may be creative or destructive, but in both cases the desire is the force urging its realization, and a person will use concentration to overcome the various obstacles in his or her path. Concentration is a powerful double-edged weapon that can cut both ways—it may protect the person or turn against him or her, depending on how it is used. Therefore we must always be aware of the real motives directing our actions and creating our problems.

"Awareness is the silent and objective observation of what is," says Krishnamurti. "In this awareness the problem unrolls itself and thus it is fully and completely understood."

The often-suggested method of self-improvement through the substitution of one emotion for another is likely to generate hypocrisy, whereas if we become deeply and honestly conscious of our shortcomings, a change of heart often takes place and transforms us almost instantly. This was true of Paul, the Apostle, of Mary Magdalen and of countless others of whom we may never have heard. This, too, is how some alcoholics give up liquor and heavy chain smokers forego their cigarettes.

An elderly woman who used to be crippled with arthritis recently told me that someone had once said to her that she would never get better so long as she continued to hate the people around her. She was intelligent enough to listen, and once she became fully aware of her faults she changed almost overnight. Before long she was able to leave her wheelchair and go back to work.

The great majority of people live in total unawareness of the real cause of their miseries, worries and unhappiness. When still in Russia and a girl in my teens, I learned an unforgettable lesson from a friend who used to write to me from a dull provincial town where his regiment was stationed. In one of his letters he said that since he had no interesting people to talk to or good books to read, he had become friends with the sun, moon, and stars, with the birds, trees, and flowers.

"Every day I talk to them and listen to their fascinating stories. And then, when we fall into silence, it seems to me that I can perceive the gentle image of Christ smiling through them to me. Thus I live in constant awareness and expectation, treating every day as though it were the last of my earthly existence. Everything then appears in a different light and acquires a greater meaning. I am never bored, lonely or unhappy: I have learned to live in the Eternal Now."

Awareness born of solitude and meditation brings a new and different understanding of life. You too may, during a quiet afternoon or evening of reflection, find that you are suddenly able to look deep down into the depths of the "inner chamber" and see yourself in a true light, "as you really are."

All of us can go through this experience and all of us can profit from it, since we know ourselves so imperfectly. Thus, for example, a despot seldom thinks he is tyrannical, a miser does not believe he is stingy, and a gossip is not aware of talking too much.

During one of my conferences someone in the audience implored me to explain the difference between prayer and mediation. In prayer one usually asks for some kind of favor or grace, thereby creating a division between the asker and the one who is being asked, between the beggar and the giver. In meditation, one does not ask for anything. In *Practical Guide for Students of Yoga*, Swami Sivananda calls meditation "the flow of continuous thought of one thing or God." It is directed to the higher being within us. In order to meditate, we must first develop the ability to concentrate to keep our minds still and steady.

The first step in concentration is the practice of Yoga postures, deep and rhythmic breathing and relaxation.

"If one doesn't have proper control over his or her own body, one cannot make proper use of the mind; one can never concentrate, much less meditate. The person who lacks mastery over his or her own physical organism cannot possibly gain spiritual consciousness; hence the need to practice posture," writes Swami Paramananda in *Concentration and Meditation*.

Since our mind is in a perpetual state of restlessness and motion, we will not manage to quiet it down without a certain amount of training. If I asked you or any other person with no previous experience to concentrate for just five minutes on a single object, you would probably find it impossible to do: your thoughts would start drifting and scattering away after the first few seconds.

Let's suppose you want to concentrate on a red rose. First you will look at it with your mind's eye, admiring its beauty, warm color and soft, velvety leaves. Then another thought will probably interfere: "How like my new velvet dress . . ." or something like that. Your thoughts soon leave the rose and drift in another direction: "That dress looked great the other night at Peter's farewell party. . . . Senseless guy, he asked me to think of him while he is in Argentina. . . . Those Argentine girls are probably going to get hold of him. . . . Peter said that Latin women make the best wives. . . . I wonder what it's like in Brazil? . . . I've heard they have beautiful beaches. . . . It's probably warm the whole year 'round. . . ." and so on and so forth until the red rose on which you started to concentrate is completely forgotten.

Something similar, with infinite variations of course, is likely to happen to almost every beginner. During the first few minutes devoted to concentration, you will have to discipline your thoughts again and again, scolding them, as if they were a small animal on a leash. As soon as you notice your thoughts beginning to stray, rein them in and return to the object of your concentration.

Every normal human being possesses the faculty of concentration, but we seldom know how to apply it consciously. Most of us use concentration automatically and instinctively. Only after we have gained command over our mental and spiritual forces will we learn to concentrate successfully.

According to my experience, the best and most suitable object of concentration for a beginner is the light of a burning candle. Before you begin, look for a quiet spot where you are not likely to be disturbed. Then choose a comfortable position in which you can sit in a relaxed way, keeping your spine straight. You may assume any of the meditative poses I have described earlier, or simply sit cross-legged. Use a chair if you prefer, but remember to keep your back straight.

Then light a candle and, your gaze fixed steadily upon the light, start on your rhythmic breathing. Look at nothing except the flame—neither the candle itself, nor the wall behind, nor any other object. Do not stare, however, and do not tense up, as you should inwardly feel completely relaxed and calm.

Let a short time pass, and then close your eyes, but continue to envision the flame with your inner eye. In other words, you must be able to see the flame constantly, even with your eyes closed. If you do not manage to keep the vision of the flame, or it vanishes too quickly, immediately reopen your eyes, look at it, then close them again. Repeat this several times until you are able to capture and hold the vision of the flame. Try to breathe rhythmically, without straining yourself.

Now begin reflecting on the qualities of the flame, upon its color and shape. Look at it with a warm feeling of affection. Ponder on its symbolical meaning as representing the eternal divine Light. Thus you are beginning to meditate on the light.

After a few days you will no longer need to light the candle. You will be able to visualize the flame by simply closing your eyes and concentrating on it. To start with, you should set aside from five to ten minutes a day for the practice of concentration.

The next stage of meditation is more difficult: Start by concentrating on the light as you have been doing so far. Then imagine that the light that you have been contemplating is no longer outside, but within you. Place it in the sacred chamber of your heart and let it shine there, illuminating every dark corner, sending out warmth and friendliness in all directions, to every living being. Let the flame in your heart grow bigger and brighter all the time, dispelling the darkness of loneliness, fear, hatred, anger, envy, jealousy, greed and lust . . . doing away with disease and pain . . . giving you health, strength and courage, becoming the source of love, compassion, and happiness.

When the light in your heart permeates your entire being and you have become one with it, you will attain a union with the eternal and divine Light, which is Love, which is Truth, which is God.

In a week or so, after you have succeeded in visualizing the candle flame without difficulty, you may change to something else or take up another object in addition to it. It is not advisable, however, to make this change before you are able to concentrate successfully or meditate on the first object you had chosen. Abandon it only when you find that it is too hard for you to hold your attention on it.

One of my students, for instance, had great difficulty in concentrating on an apple because after visualizing it he instinctively felt like eating it. In a case like this, one should not insist. Dismiss the object and replace it with another one, but always choose something beautiful and pleasant on which to concentrate.

When you notice you are making good progress, you may start concentrating and meditating on abstract matters, on different values and diverse qualities and ideas. But be extremely careful in choosing only those that are positive, right, noble and inspirational.

"We must not remain content with lower forms of concentration," writes Swami Paramananda. "These may bring us physical health, prosperity or success, because concentration always gives power; but even though we acquire more wealth, greater honor or increase bodily strength, we shall find that one part of our being still remains unsatisfied in spite of all our worldly acquisitions. Never will it be content until we awaken and begin to work for our higher development."

As concentration gives added power, we should be very careful in choosing what we want, so that we do not concentrate on the fulfillment of base or selfish desires.

It is not always easy to determine whether our wish is selfish or not. Is the wish to be healthy, for instance, a selfish one? Is the desire to marry a person you love selfish?

Therefore, when you make a wish, you should always add "if it is right for me." By doing so, we do not impose our will upon the Higher Will. In other words, we are saying, "Thy will be done." But if we are bent on getting what we want, we may find eventually that it was the worse thing that could have happened to us; we simply didn't know it at the time we were in pursuit of it.

It is only through proper and unselfish meditation that the student can finally enter the temple of the undistracted and abstract mind, and in silence and solitude come to the realization of the One Ultimate Reality and reach the peace beyond all understanding.

Appendix I • A Guide to Diet and Recipes

Many of my students and readers have begged me to outline a diet for them. As I have already pointed out in Lesson Two, this is difficult to do since food requirements and tastes vary not only with the individual but also with one's age. Here follows an example of my personal diet, which would hardly satisfy most people, partly because I am a vegetarian and partly because I take only one meal a day—for breakfast and dinner I eat very little.

Upon getting up: A glass of water that has been kept overnight in a copper tumbler, taken with or without lemon

Breakfast: A cup of soybean milk or cereal coffee
Some almonds and raisins
A grapefruit or orange

Between meals: Plenty of water, some fresh fruit and vegetable juices, and ripe fruit in season

Lunch: Soup
Green salad with or without dressing
1 cooked vegetable or 1 raw vegetable or a

serving of any one of the following: bean stew/
bean sprouts, brown rice, semolina or peeled
oats, or a potato/baked potato with oil or
butter and soybean sauce or vegetable salt
(the skin of the potato is included)

Dinner: A cup of cereal coffee with honey
A sliced tomato with cheese, or one yogurt
with honey and wheat germ, or a slice of whole
wheat bread with avocado and vegetable salt

Before going to bed: A glass of water

About Dr. William Howard Hay's diet, the Hay diet, which has been brought again to the public's attention, I have received repeated requests to explain it. This diet classifies food so that carbohydrates are separated from proteins and from acid- and sulfur-content foods; they should not be eaten together at any one meal. The reason is that alkaline-forming foods and acid-forming foods each require different conditions for their proper digestion.

Starch should be well chewed so that it may be converted into glucose by the saliva before it leaves the mouth to reach the stomach, where it lies almost inactive until it passes through the duodenum into the intestine where digestion continues. Protein, on the contrary, is digested mainly in the stomach, where gastric juices begin to secrete as soon as the protein reaches it. If carbohydrates are present in the stomach at the same time, they start fermenting because the acid in the gastric juices affects the starch, thereby creating gas and acidity. The same thing happens when starch is eaten together with foods containing acid, such as lemons and other citrus fruits, tomatoes or vinegar, or when eaten with sulfurous food such as cabbage, peas, beans, cauliflower, brussels sprouts or eggs. This classification of foods is especially beneficial for people suffering from indigestion and gas.

The Hay Diet Food Classification

A	B

A

PROTEINS
Brains
Cheese
Clams
Crabs
Eggs
Fish
Gelatin
Low-fat or skim milk
Meat
Milk
Nuts
Oysters

FRUITS
Apples
Apricots
Berries
Cherries
Currants
Grapefruit
Grapes
Kumquats
Lemons
Limes
Mangoes
Oranges
Peaches
Pears

B

STARCH
Artichokes
Chestnuts (cooked)
Corn
Cornstarch
Oatmeal
Pastries and cakes
Popcorn
Potatoes
Refined cereals
Sauces with white flour
Soups with white flour thickening
Spaghetti
Tapioca
White bread
White flour
White rice
Whole grain bread
Whole grain cereals
Whole grain flour
Whole wheat rice

SWEETS
Candy
Ice cream (commercial)
Jams and jellies
Jell-O
Preserves
Stewed fruit

(The items in italics are not recommended at all.)

A

Pineapple
Plums
Pomegranates
Prunes
Raisins
Tangerines
Tomatoes

ROOTS

Beets
Cabbage
Carrots
Celery
Parsnips
Radishes
Turnips

SALADS AND LETTUCE

(all kinds)
Chicory
Chives
Cucumber
Garlic
Onions (green)
Parsley
Watercress

NEUTRAL

Artichokes (cone)
Asparagus

B

Syrup (refined)
White sugar

FATS

(No more than three in one meal)
Avocado
Butter
Coconut
Cream
Egg yolks
Fats (animal)
Lard
Nuts
Oils

SUGARS

(not more than two in one meal)
Bananas
Dates
Figs
Honey
Maple sugar
Maple syrup
Persimmons
Prunes
Raisins
Sugar (raw, brown)

(The items in italics are not recommended at all.)

A

Beans (dried, green*, snap*)
Beet tops
Broccoli*
Brussels sprouts*
Cabbage
Cauliflower*
Celery
Chard
Corn (tender)
Dandelion greens
Eggplant
Kale
Kraut
Leeks
Lentils*
Lettuce
Lima beans (green)*
Mushrooms
Okra
Onions*
Peas (dried, green*)
Peppers (green)
Pumpkin
Spinach
Squash
Vegetable marrow

Items marked with an asterisk may be eaten together with salads, vegetables or fruit as a main course, in any amount, as long as no other proteins or starches are included. They are not recommended for people suffering from gas. Cabbage should not be eaten by people troubled by indigestion.

As already mentioned, no cooked sulfur foods such as cabbage, cauliflower, turnips, peas, beans, etc., are to be combined with starches, as this produces gas.

Lean meat, game, poultry, liver, kidneys, heart, sweetbreads, and fish may be eaten prepared in any way except fried or with the addition of breadcrumbs, sauces, and gravies thickened with flour.

Cleansing Diet

There are several good ways to cleanse the system. One way is to stay from five to ten days on a mono diet, that is, to eat as much as one likes of any one of the following:

a) Watermelon: especially good for cleansing the kidneys. If you feel too hungry, eat a slice of whole wheat bread or whole-wheat wafers.

b) Grated raw apples and herb tea with lemon—especially good for people suffering from dysentery, colitis or diarrhea. (The apples should be grated on plastic, glass or stainless-steel graters.)

c) Fresh grapes, unsprayed with chemical products, to avoid danger of poisoning. This mono diet is beneficial for the liver.

d) Coconut water only—cleanses the liver and alkalizes the system.

e) Grapefruit and/or orange juice or both: alkalizes the system.

One of my students, who owns a garden where she grows her own vegetables and fruit, sent me a less rigid cleansing diet. She was able to overcome a critical asthmatic condition by practicing the breathing exercises and the Yoga postures, in addition to keeping the following diet:

Health Diet

On arising: A glass of water with fresh lemon juice

Breakfast: Any herb tea or coffee substitute or raw cow's,
                     goat's (better) or soybean milk, 1 slice whole
                     grain bread sweetened with honey or date or
                     raw sugar, or 1 slice whole grain bread with
                     date or almond butter or small dish of stewed
                     fruit or any fresh fruit in season

Between meals: Water
                     Fruit or vegetable juice or fruit eaten out of hand

Lunch: Low-fat/skim milk, or herb tea or cereal coffee
                     Salad made with any raw greens, including
                     watercress and parsley especially, with a dressing
                     made from the juice of 1 lemon, vegetable salt,
                     and safflower, sunflower, sesame or soybean oil
                     1 slice whole grain bread or baked potato
                     Yogurt or cottage cheese or sour cream
                     with any fruit

Dinner: Herb tea or cereal coffee
                     Vegetable broth
                     Celery sticks, carrots and sliced cucumbers
                     1 serving of meat, fish, poultry, cheese,
                     eggs or nuts
                     1 serving of a vegetable grown above ground
                     1 serving of a vegetable grown below ground
                     Fresh fruit or stewed fruit or raisins and nuts

Take a spoonful of safflower, sunflower, sesame, or cod liver oil, four
hours after your last meal.

Reducing Diet

On arising: A glass of water with fresh lemon juice

Lunch: Salad without any dressing except lemon juice
1 cup of soup (no cream, butter or flour)
1 soft boiled egg or soybean cake or tofu, or
3 1/2 oz. of lean meat or cooked, baked or
roasted fish
Celery sticks, raw carrots, radishes,
cucumbers, etc.
Fruit in season
Skim or low-fat milk, 8 fl. oz.

Dinner: 1 cup of soup
1 boiled egg or piece of cheese
1/2 cup serving of vegetable
Salad (no dressing except lemon juice)
Skim milk, 8 fl. oz., or yogurt
1/2 cup serving of fruit.
Herb tea or cereal coffee with skim milk
(no cream or sugar)

Evening snack: Any kind of fresh fruit, fruit juice, or
vegetable juice

Diet for People over Thirty-five

Our body reaches its full maturity around the age of twenty-eight. By the time we reach thirty-five, it starts to gradually decrease its activities and the life processes begin to slow down their pace. Therefore, if we want to remain healthy and young it is unavoidable to make certain changes in our diet and eating habits so as not to overburden the digestive system with an extra effort.

After the age of thirty-five, we should start cutting down on all saturated fats (such as lard, bacon, butter, nuts) and refined carbohydrates (such as bread, pastry, pies, spaghetti, and other products containing white flour and white sugar). We should eliminate them completely by the age of sixty, after which even eggs and potatoes should be eaten sparingly. The same is true of all other starchy and sulfurous foods that create gas when eaten together during the same meal. (See in this same appendix the Hay diet food classification.)

Fried food is never good for anyone and should be given up completely after the age of thirty-five. The food we eat should be steamed or boiled, baked or broiled. Raw foods such as fruit and vegetables may be juiced or processed, if desired.

A glass of water with lemon juice every morning and a pint of low-fat milk a day should never be omitted. The following are the foods recommended for people over thirty-five: low-fat milk, cottage cheese, soybean products (milk, cheese), fish, shrimps, oysters, lean meat, alfalfa sprouts, bell peppers, carrots and carrot juice, fresh corn, dandelions, endive, parsley, romaine, and watercress. Included also are foods that contain vitamins, minerals and protein in abundance, such as grapefruits, oranges, lemons, apricots, grapes, figs, dates, raisins, plums, prunes, boysenberries, strawberries, raspberries, cantaloupe, watermelon and papayas.

One of the best alkalizing drinks is potato water, which helps the system get rid of toxins. People suffering from arthritis are especially benefited by drinking potato water first thing in the morning, at least once during the day, and the last thing at night. They should also eat one or two baked potatoes, skin included, every day. They may be added to salads, soups or vegetables directly before serving.

The Indians claim that people afflicted with arthritis should always keep a raw unpeeled winter-crop potato close to their skin. As soon as it turns too hard or too soft, it should be discarded and replaced by a fresh one. I myself have seen a woman who previously had hardly been able to move her fingers open and close her fists a week after she started playing around with a potato. She kept it in her apron pocket during the day, holding it in her hands whenever she had the chance. At night, to prevent the potato from rolling, she slipped her hand, with the potato in it, into a stocking.

Since there is no risk of any kind involved in holding a potato, and since you may even start a new fashion by wearing one around the neck like a medallion, you could safely try this experiment. Just be sure to remember that the potato must be a winter-crop one. And let me know the results.

Recipes

SALADS

One head romaine lettuce or any other green salad plus watercress, parsley, tomatoes, green onions, chopped celery, fresh cucumber, finely cut bell peppers, alfalfa sprouts or bean sprouts, any herb, mint leaves, grated carrots or grated beets, in any combination desired sunflower seeds or piñon nuts to taste (1 to 2 heaping tablespoons).

Combine the above ingredients, breaking the salad into small pieces by hand. Directly before serving, add any of the following dressings:

(a) Lemon juice, oil, soybean sauce or vegetable salt, honey, Sesame Tahini (available in health food stores), in any combination to taste. The general rule is about 2 parts oil to 1 part lemon juice.

(b) Sour cream with honey water

(c) Oil, lemon, grated Roquefort cheese, in any combination desired

(d) Egg yolk, lemon juice, salt, honey, in any combination desired

(e) Low-fat milk, grated onion, vegetable salt, a dash of curry powder

SOUPS

Cauliflower Soup
1 medium cauliflower
1 medium onion, chopped
1 medium carrot, diced
6 cups water
3 laurel leaves
Soybean sauce to taste
Seasoning to taste

Boil carrot and bay leaves for about 15 minutes. Add cauliflower, cut up into flowerets, and the chopped onion. Simmer, covered, until cauliflower is tender. Remove laurel leaves. Season and serve. Serves 4 liberally.

Spinach Soup

1 package chopped spinach
1 large carrot
1 medium onion, finely chopped
1 medium potato (optional)
4 cups water
3 laurel leaves
Juice of 1/2 lemon
Seasoning to taste
Hard-cooked eggs, 1 per serving

Except lemon juice, simmer all ingredients together, tightly covered, for about half an hour. Add lemon juice and seasoning. Serve with sliced hard-cooked eggs. Serves 4 generously.

Carrot Soup

4 medium carrots
1 large onion
4 cups water
2 laurel leaves
1 tablespoon oil or butter
Seasoning to taste
Chopped parsley for garnish

Combine all ingredients, bring to a boil and simmer, tightly covered, until vegetables are tender. Sprinkle with fresh parsley. Serves 4 generously.

Pea Soup
3/4 package split peas
1 whole large onion
1 medium onion, chopped and sautéed in a little oil
6 cups water
3 laurel leaves
Seasoning to taste

Combine all ingredients, except sautéed onion; bring to a boil and simmer, covered, for about an hour or until peas are soft. Remove laurel leaves and the whole onion. Add the cooked chopped onion and simmer a few minutes longer. Season to taste. Serves 4 generously.

ELECTRIC BLENDER RECIPES
Soups may also be made by using an electric blender. These soups will be ready within 10 to 15 minutes. Here are some recipes for such soups:

Carrot Soup:
4 medium carrots
1 large onion
1 laurel leaf
4 cups water
Seasoning to taste

Cut up onion and carrot and boil with laurel leaf for 5 to 6 minutes. Remove laurel leaf. Allow to cool off, then put in blender and mix for 2 to 3 minutes. Cook on low flame for another 5 minutes. Season to taste. Add a little oil or butter if desired. Serves 4.

The above recipe may be varied according to your own preference. Here are a few suggestions:

Celery and Leek Soup
1/4 bunch celery, broken into small pieces, with strings removed
2 leeks, cut into pieces
1 medium potato
4 cups water
Seasoning to taste

Proceed as for Carrot Soup made in blender. Serves 4.

Potato Soup
2 medium potatoes, diced
1 onion, diced
4 cups water
1 laurel leaf (optional)
1 to 2 tablespoons oil or butter
Seasoning to taste

Proceed as for Carrot Soup made in blender. Serves 4.

Cauliflower Soup
1 small cauliflower
1 onion
4 cups water
1 laurel leaf (optional)
Seasoning to taste

Proceed as for Carrot Soup made in blender. Serves 4.

VARIOUS DISHES

Cauliflower Casserole

1 large cauliflower
2 medium onions, sautéed in a little oil
3 tablespoons grated Parmesan or Cheddar cheese
1 cup thin white sauce, with a little tomato sauce added
Seasoning to taste

Cut cauliflower into small flowerets and boil, covered, in a little water until nearly done. Reserve water. Cover bottom of a Pyrex dish with the cooked onions and arrange cauliflower over them. Make white sauce, using the water in which cauliflower was boiled. Add tomato sauce to taste. Pour over cauliflower, sprinkle with cheese and dot with butter. Bake in 375° oven for 20 to 30 minutes. Serves 4 to 6.

Soybean Milk

3/4 cups soybeans, soaked overnight
2 cups water
1 teaspoon salt
1 1/2 tablespoons brown sugar
3 cups water

In an electric blender, combine the soaked beans with 2 cups of water and blend at medium speed for 2 minutes. Pour into saucepan; add salt and brown sugar; bring to a boil, stirring constantly, and simmer for about 2 minutes. Strain, reserving residue. Return residue to saucepan, add 3 more cups of water, and repeat the process. Strain again and add this second batch of liquid to the first. If too thick, dilute with a little water. Keep in refrigerator. Shake before using. Yield: 5 cups.

Spinach Soufflé:
2 packages spinach
1 or 2 tablespoons dry mushrooms, soaked in water for 1/2 hour, or
an equivalent amount of fresh mushrooms
2 eggs, separated
3 tablespoons grated cheese
1/2 cup hot milk
Seasoning to taste
Dash of nutmeg
1 clove garlic, finely chopped
Soy oil

Boil spinach, drain well and chop coarsely. Combine egg yolks with
milk, taking care not to curdle, and cook over very low heat, stirring
constantly, until mixture begins to thicken. Add to spinach. Season to
taste with salt and nutmeg.

Cut up mushrooms and sauté in soy oil with the chopped garlic for 5
to 10 minutes. Add to spinach. Whip egg whites very stiff and fold
into the mixture. Pour into casserole and bake in 375° oven for about
30 minutes. Serves 4 to 6.

Mushroom Sauce
1/2 lb. fresh mushrooms or 1 1/2 ounces dry mushrooms
1 tablespoon cooking oil
1 medium onion, finely chopped
1 clove garlic, finely chopped
Salt and pepper to taste
Sour cream to taste
Chopped parsley for garnish

If dry mushrooms are used, cover and soak in water for half an hour.
Reserve water. Chop mushrooms but do not peel. Sauté onion and

garlic in oil until transparent, add mushrooms and continue cooking over low flame, covered, until mushrooms are limp—about 10 minutes. Add a little of the water in which mushrooms have soaked to make a sauce. Season to taste, add sour cream and let bubble up. Simmer another 5 to 6 minutes. Add fresh parsley last.

Sauerkraut Salad

1 lb. fresh sauerkraut
1 medium apple, diced
1 small onion, finely chopped
1 heaping tablespoon caraway seeds
2 to 3 tablespoons cooking oil
1 teaspoon honey

Sprinkle sauerkraut with caraway seeds. Add oil and honey, mix thoroughly and let stand at least half an hour, so that seeds will soften. Add chopped apple and mix again. Serves 4 to 6.

Carrot-Rice-Nut Loaf

4 whole eggs, lightly beaten
5 tablespoons vegetable oil
1 teaspoon vegetable salt
3 cups grated carrots
2 cups cooked brown rice
2 cups chopped walnuts
1 medium onion, chopped
1 green pepper, chopped (optional)

Combine eggs, oil and salt until thoroughly blended. Add other ingredients and mix thoroughly. Pour into lightly greased casserole, press down lightly, and bake in 375° oven for 30 minutes. Serves 6.

Eggplant Steaks

1 large eggplant, cut into 1/2-inch slices

Salt and pepper to taste

Butter

Season eggplant slices, dot each with butter and arrange in broiler. Broil under medium flame until tender. Serves 4.

Spinach and Rice Ring

2 packages spinach, cooked and chopped

3/4 cup milk

2 whole eggs, lightly beaten

1 1/2 cups cooked brown rice

1 small onion, grated

Dash of nutmeg (optional)

Seasoning to taste

Mix all ingredients together, adding milk and beaten egg last. Bake in 400° oven for 30 minutes. Serves 4.

Appendix II • Letters and E-Mails to the Author and to the Indra Devi Foundation

Publisher's note: The following are but a few of the letters and E-mails in praise of Indra Devi's popular and effective method of teaching Yoga, and in appreciation of her first book, *Forever Young, Forever Healthy*.

TEL AVIV, ISRAEL

Dear Indra Devi:

There are no words to tell you what Yoga has done for us. I simply do not know what would have happened to us without it, for it has brought not only happiness but an entirely new existence.

The Headstand and other exercises actually saved my husband's life when he was suffering a severe form of nervous depression.

I am unspeakably happy to have had the chance to study Yoga with you. My husband and I are able to teach it to other people and help them. Both of us and our students are eagerly awaiting the publication of your new book.

With all best wishes,
Raya Riskin

Dear Indra Devi:

This is just a line to let you know how much I have enjoyed your book *Forever Young, Forever Healthy*. It agrees in every respect with our own philosophy of life. I have studied Yoga before, but never realized the importance of the various headstands and exercises, as I was more into weight lifting and other strenuous sports. However, I am adding your exercises to the barbell and must say they are great.

As you say, they are not for the tender ones who do not have the courage to start up on such rigorous discipline. They have only themselves to blame for a feeble, senile, foggy-brained old age, and plenty of doctor's bills.

Yours truly,
Robert G. Collier

Dearest Teacher:

Yoga does not need me to enhance its values, except for those who think that miracles do happen without effort and faith.

As you know, X-rays of my spine showed several calcium deposits. These were caused by two severe car accidents and a fall which worsened my critical condition, and made an abdominal operation necessary.

The Yoga exercises you taught me, together with my continuous efforts of following them at home, not only have completely healed my spine but have erased all trace of scars. I have recovered full use of the intestinal tract together with the natural functions of muscles atrophied by adhesions formed after the operations.

I have regained full coordination and use of movements for dancing. With the restoration of my physical health, my creative energies have been channeled into a new field—I started clay modeling for my own enjoyment and am already exhibiting now.

My own father-in-law, who is a doctor, was delighted at my finding a true teacher of Yoga who has me convinced of continuously practicing her teachings in order to keep me always in good health.

As ever,
Manuella

POST OFFICE, ENTUMENI
ZULULAND, SOUTH AFRICA

My dear Madam Devi:

Not so long ago, I came across your article on deep breathing where-upon I immediately ordered your book. Its clear, simple and intelligent approach to Yoga impressed me so much that it prompted me to write you. I decided to order a supply so that people here could get their copy without too much delay. It may please you to know that you have already acquired many ardent followers here in South Africa.

I am so thankful to say that the dull pain on my left side, in the kidney region, has subsided, and I feel so much better for doing the rhythmic breathing exercises for a few minutes twice a day. I am timing them to my walking pace when going to my office (I am an engineer here and live within walking distance). I have found that my eyesight is better although I have been taking the exercises for only eleven weeks.

Let me congratulate you and thank you for writing such a splendid and useful book. It has become a textbook for most Yoga teachers here.

Yours sincerely,
Cecil F. Wickes

ENNIS, TEXAS

Dear Indra Devi:

I am a Methodist minister, seventy-two years of age. I suffered from sciatic rheumatism several years ago, and it left a stiffness in my limbs, particularly my knees. I did not realize how great that stiffness was until I began your exercises. But, best of all, I never knew what complete relief was until I learned to relax the bones of the spine and pelvis through your Yoga exercises.

I began attempting to practice some of the simpler ones and, to my amazement, just a few minutes spent at them seemed to give me a wonderful "lift" both physically and mentally.

I am really convinced of the merits of this system, and intend to do the exercises more regularly.

My elimination is so much better, also the terrible bloating and dizziness after meals. My general health and well-being have greatly improved thanks to you.

It is my sincere belief that if I had known and practiced the principles of Yoga many years ago, I could have enjoyed not only a higher degree of good health, but could have given better service to God and man. I should say that Yoga is proving that Occidentals have much to learn from the Orientals, who have steadfastly practiced these health-building principles for hundreds of years.

With kindest regards to you and sincere appreciation of the service you are rendering to suffering people.

I am gratefully yours,
Roy A. Langston
Pastor, First Methodist Church

BOMBAY, INDIA

Dear Mataji Indra Devi:

You no doubt already know the good news that the Sindhi translation of your book has received an award from our government. We are all very happy and proud of you.

Your book has made even us Indians more keenly aware of the great benefits of the Yoga Asanas. You have rendered a great service to humanity by writing it. You would be surprised to know how many people here have benefited by following your instructions. One of our close friends, for example, the wife of a university professor, suffered for many years from nervous stomach troubles, arthritis, and female disorders. After a few months of practicing Yoga and following your diet, she has completely recovered from all her troubles and feels like a different person now.

Books are my hobby: you know that I am the first man to have published in pictures our sacred Bhagavat Gita. Allow me to congratulate and thank you for having written such a precious and useful book.

Your sincere friend,
Parmanand S. Mehra

Dear Miss Devi:

May I express my heart-felt and deepest admiration for your work?

I am thirty years old, and a professional musician. I have also been an alcoholic for eleven years.

Since practicing the Yoga postures diligently for the past few months, following the diet you outlined in your book, and sleeping on a hard surface, I have achieved the following results:

1) I have given up alcohol and no longer have any desire for it.

2) I have also lost interest in smoking, soft drinks, and spicy foods, something which I never dreamed possible.

3) I have lost much of my excess weight, am less nervous and depressed.

4) There have been remarkable improvements in my health: my liver condition and my ulcerative colitis are much better.

My friends are amazed at the changes Yoga has brought about in me. I want to continue progress in this wonderful gift to mankind and would like to help others someday.

Thank you, and may the Higher Self smile on you forever.

T. N.

Dear Indra Devi:

I have your book *Forever Young, Forever Healthy,* translated into Japanese, and am very pleased with it.

I am thirty-eight years old and have suffered great pains due to a nervous heart condition. Since I started on the Yoga postures, my pains have decreased greatly. My wife, thirty-two years old, has found the exercises of much help in losing weight, and my five-year-old son has no more asthma trouble since the day he began exercising. I also have a daughter, and both children have had a lot of trouble with tonsillitis, but, thanks to the Lion Posture, their sore throats are much better. Our family has found the Yoga exercises very useful for promoting better elimination.

Yours very truly,
R. T.

BAD HOMBURG, GERMANY

Much esteemed Miss Indra Devi:

Your kind letter arrived on Christmas day and I must tell you that it was my best Christmas present.

I am so glad that you have decided to write another book and to include in it suggestions for concentration and meditation.

You are such a good teacher that it is almost impossible to make a mistake when following your instructions.

Personally, I am of the opinion that your book is the best one on Yoga. I have read a number of them but none is as clear and practical as yours.

I want to report to you that we are all working diligently and I am making steady progress with the Lotus Pose and other postures, although I am still far from perfection. The Headstand is priceless and its results are outstanding. The Yoga exercises are remarkable: The fat ones get slimmer and the thin ones gain weight and get stronger; constipation disappears, the body becomes elastic and the spirits brighten up.

I am a seeker and you have given me so much.
Wishing you everything good,
I am always at your service,
A. G.

Dear Indra Devi:

It is with great pleasure that I write to you, distinguished and renowned Yoga expert, in order to express my heartfelt gratitude for the personal training I received, upon your trip to Mexico City.

This letter would require great length if I were to describe the numerous benefits that the practice of the postures and rhythmic deep breathing, as well as the meditation, concentration and relaxation, have brought to me.

I wish to inform you that I am intensely happy for my increased ability to carry out my work as an air pilot, which reflects in my greater resistance to fatigue and an increased control of the constant nervous tension that occurs during operational flights, as well as better judgment to evaluate situations, both when at work, and beyond my duties.

I should add that doctors, psychiatrists, physiologists, and psychologists all agree that the fundamental qualities every pilot should develop are: a perfect psychic balance, good emotional stability and control over one's self that allows to keep calm in difficult situations. That is why I trust myself completely to recommend Yoga as a valuable aid in perfecting the pilot's training, offering a long professional life, in use of all physical, psychic and intellectual faculties.

Your grateful student,
Enrique Sáenz de Sicilia I
Air Pilot Captain

SAN PEDRO, BUENOS AIRES, ARGENTINA

Dear Mataji:

We are grateful to God from the bottom of our hearts for granting us the opportunity to meet you.

The times spent together with you in San Pedro remain unforgettable and full of feelings unknown to us, to the point where our group defines this period as "before Mataji and after Mataji—this last full of love and light."

Next month we will organize our work in order to give Yoga lessons to the children in the D. F. Sarmiento Institute you visited.

Your conference at the Municipality was so precise that even those who ignored what Yoga was felt the current of your wisdom.

Let me tell you a short story: a young single woman, who had never really accepted her maternity, bought your cassette and, together with her five-year-old daughter, meditated with the candle and listened to your words. The next day was Mother's Day, and she was able to experience that full and joyful love for the first time in her life.

We take leave of you, wishing that our group remain in your heart, just as you remain in ours.

May God bless you,
YOGA OM Group

POSADAS, MISIONES, ARGENTINA

Dear most beautiful Mataji:

It is not easy to write when your right hand is in a cast. But so great is the need of communicating with you, that here I am.

I need to tell you how wonderful it has been to know you, to receive the rays of your intense light and to share your peace, harmony and love.

Your visit to Posadas was like a fairy tale. A fairy tale that transformed us. And I am not exaggerating when I assure you that we still feel you here among us. Besides often remembering you, we feel you almost physically, going up and down the stairs, and giving us an example of peacefulness.

I wish to personally express to you that our meeting together has been like going back to an old house where there is always a warm fire and the love of friends awaiting us; that is, a temporary shelter to stop for a while and then continue with a firmer step walking toward the Real and Absolute One.

Dear Mataji, with the memory of the songs we sang together,
I remain, full of love,
Olga Kolesnikoff

Congratulations for this site. I had the opportunity of attending the (Yoga) Convention some weeks ago and even though I don't know much about this discipline, I am deeply grateful for having such a wonderful experience. Today, when violence, negativity, lack of values, envy and pain are everywhere, I was able to go beyond, to a different world—one of love, peace and harmony, of which I did not want to awaken. Again, thank you for everything. All the best, Juan Carlos.

Juan Carlos Hernández, Olavarría, Bs. As., Argentina

I learned what Yoga is through the books by Indra Devi, a being full of light. I felt compelled to practice this wonderful discipline that brought on many positive changes in myself, such as the awakening of my conscience. I started to understand the meaning of life, and to grow in a spiritual direction. I am no longer as high-strung as I used to be and I let things happen to me, without planning them. Thank you for being there and offering us your Love and Light. Mónica.

Mónica Arruti de Zunino, Jesús María, Córdoba, Argentina

Since my divorce, I have been going through some of the most difficult moments in my life, yet Yoga has helped me to start growing. I felt the need to continue enriching myself, so I searched for a Yoga site on the Web, and what a wonderful surprise to be here, reading your stories and messages, which right now give a soft little rub to my heart. Thanks a million.

Teresa Rodríguez Jiménez, Colombia

I am from Venezuela and have lived here in Miami for four years. I have read several of Mataji's books, which have helped me in my spiritual growth. My wife Laura is a Yoga instructor and I have been practicing it regularly every day for the last year, with incredible results. I feel physically younger and calmer and my level of tolerance has greatly increased. As Mataji, I too have been in India (. . .), an unforgettable experience that changed my life. . . . Thank you and Namaste.

Alejandro Galavis, Miami, FL, USA.

Dear Iana and David: I don't know how to express my gratitude for the orientation, wise leadership and kindness with which you shower your teachings on us. You have allowed me to grow spiritually and to help people who have come to me for help. Both my life as well as theirs have changed for the better. They say that wherever there is a person who meditates, violence ceases all around. That is why I believe it is very important to go deep into meditation, one of the most difficult tasks of all. All my best to you, Octavio.

Octavio Lecaros Palma, Punta Arenas, Chile

Dear Mataji, Iana and David: I love finding a Yoga Web site that is so complete, and to know that there are more and more people interested in this practice. We have to help let others to know about it—friends, colleagues, family, because, as Mataji Indra Devi says, it really changes your life and helps you leave behind a negative approach and focus on good feelings, sharing them with everyone else. Thank you Mataji Indra Devi for your teachings and wisdom. Thank you Iana and David Lifar for helping to make Yoga known. With love,

Francoise Brailovsky, México, D.F., México

My friend picked up a *Yoga* magazine in the health food store and when I looked over her shoulder at it, there was a beautiful picture of Indra Devi. I was so excited! I read *Yoga for Americans* over 30 years ago when I was a school girl. I lost my original copy and bought another one years ago. Her work introduced me to Yoga, meditation, chakras, and Eastern philosophical thought. Many times, when I'd feel "stuck" in my life, I'd pull out her book and it would bring me back to basics. I've been a herbalist now for 23 years and she remains a wonderful inspiration to me. Where may I obtain a better copy of the beautiful photo that was in the magazine? Thank you!

Carol McGrath, Victoria, B.C. Canada

Dear Iana and David: I was a student at the Foundation and for lack of time, I now do Yoga on my own, but assisted by an instructor from the Foundation, as I would never be able to do Yoga with anyone else that is not connected to your Center. I was lucky to receive Mataji's embrace once; she is a being full of Light. The Web site is very interesting. Thanks.

Cecilia Tofanari, Buenos Aires, Argentina